MOVE IT
LIKE YOU MEAN IT

A Quiet Word About Parkinson's Disease In Men

Henri 'RENOIR' Rennie

Cartoons by Angus Gardner

1

Thank you to Meredith for love, encouragement and support,

and to everyone involved in

www.moveit4parkinsons.com

who inspired this book.

MEREDIAN
PICTURES & WORDS

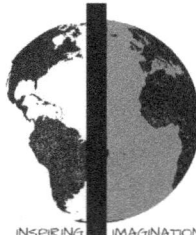

INSPIRING IMAGINATION

By the same author:

Mid-Life Crisis MANagement: A Quiet Word About Surviving Middle Age and Male Menopause

Praise for *Mid-Life Crisis MANagement*:

"It is not uncommon for middle-aged men to ignore and neglect their health. This lack of attention often means that men present with advanced disease that could have been identified and managed earlier if medical attention had been sought. Improved physical and mental condition with advancing age is a clear benefit for men who pay attention to their health care needs. This book identifies the key issues in men's health that should be addressed if one is seeking an optimal quality of life with advancing age. I strongly recommend that men read and take notice of its messages."

Professor Darrell Crawford MD FRACP
Head of The School of Medicine, University of Queensland
Director of Research, Gallipoli Medical Research Foundation
Practising Gastroenterologist

Table of Contents

About the Author

Who is Henri Rennie, anyway?

I'm not a doctor. Or a psychologist. Or any sort of professional New Age therapist, though I've studied a fair bit. I'm a bloke who asks questions, and writes down the answers in a way that other blokes will understand.

For a long time I've been interested in health and healing. I've done First Aid and Lifesaving Certificates, training in Occupational Health & Safety, a Certificate in Reiki and been trained as a Nutrition Advisor at the Sanoviv Medical Institute in Baja California.

I've turned my hand at a lot of jobs over the years. At various times I've been an actor, a barman, a journo, and coached a (pretty ordinary) soccer team. I've sung in a 70's suburban rock band, and been a greenkeeper, a plumber's mate, a Public Servant, a security guard, even a vacuum cleaner salesman.

I've worked in offices and pubs, on building sites and on the road, in colleges and in jail.

Along the way I've probably eaten and drunk more than I should have, and exercised less than was good for me. I've had what feels like a filing cabinet full of my own health issues. Lots of the common ones – broken legs, kidney stones, asthma and pneumonia, heart attack, and some less common – busted spine, three types of arthritis all at once, some of my guts removed.

Family, friends and acquaintances have likewise been through a bunch of stuff. Some survived, others didn't.

But I've been lucky – I've survived, and learned as I went along.

These days I travel quite a bit, talking to people and trying to learn stuff as I go. Mostly I write.

I've learned a lot of facts, looked at statistics, gathered some opinions and formed some of my own. And now I'm sharing that with you.

Sometimes I'm known as 'Renoir' when I'm writing fiction, or drawing cartoons.

But this is another part of me. This part wants to do more than make people laugh. This part sees blokes suffering, often (not always) in silence and wants to do something to help. The *Quiet Word* books are my way of trying to do that.

Blokes don't often talk face to face – we talk better shoulder to shoulder. That's why we have better conversations in the car or standing at the bar than over the dinner table.

Even then, there's a lot we don't talk much about out loud, even to our mates. Like our health. Think of this book as a quiet word – a quiet word that might save your life.

.oOo.

INTRODUCTION: Why This Book?

I'm a big boxing fan. The late great Muhammad Ali at his best remains one of the greatest fighters I've ever seen – far and away the best heavyweight. But my clearest, most inspiring memory doesn't come from any of his bouts.

It's that shaking hand lighting the Olympic flame in Atlanta in July 1996.

Ali was diagnosed with Parkinson's Disease in 1984. He'd probably already had the disease for at least four years by then, and he had it until his death 32 years later.

When he came out for that Olympic moment, in front of millions of viewers all over the world, he said, "I have Parkinson's Disease but Parkinson's Disease doesn't have me."[1]

He made that point over and over again in interviews and public appearances for the best part of another two decades.

Much more recently I was playing bowls with a bloke who sadly said to me over a beer afterwards, "I'm gonna have to give the game away."

"Why?" I asked. "You're playing alright. Better than I am, though that's not saying much."

"Ah, the doc says I've got Parkinson's. So that's it. It's only gonna get worse – all downhill from here."

Since then I've met quite a few people with PD (as it's sometimes called), and others actively involved in helping them: doctors and therapists of different types. One message keeps coming back. Parkinson's may not be curable (yet) but it *is* manageable. That was Ali's message. Parkinson's Disease *can* be faced with courage, grace and humour. There is hope.

It takes some effort, and some persistence, but if you actually enjoy your life and want to continue doing so, I reckon it's worth it.

As with anything medical, there's a lot of jargon out there about Parkinson's. And as blokes, we're not always very good at admitting we don't completely understand what a doctor or specialist or whatever is trying to tell us. So I've tried to make it simple. There's detail in this book, but feel free to skim through that if the 'sciencey stuff' doesn't interest you. Find what you actually need.

Sooner or later you really *do* have to talk to someone about what you're going through, and if this book can help you to know what you (and they) are talking about, then it's done its job, and I'll be happy!

Cheers,
Renoir

1 WHAT IS PARKINSON'S DISEASE?

The technical description of Parkinson's Disease is that it's a "neurode-generative brain disorder".

That means that there are cells in the brain that stop working properly. They're cells that produce something called dopamine. Dopamine does a lot of good things for the body, one of the most important of which is making sure that the body's movements are smooth and controlled. (It's also involved in the ability to feel pleasure – more on that later.)

When there isn't enough dopamine in the body then movements get out of control – either too much (tremors and twitches), or too little (stiffness or even paralysis).

It's a lot more common than you might think, too. There are around 110,000 people in Australia who live with Parkinson's. That's around one in every three hundred, and about 38 more are diagnosed every day.

Let's put that in perspective. PD is more commonly diagnosed than well known and better publicized nasties such as:
- Breast cancer;
- Colon cancer;
- Stomach cancer;
- Pancreatic cancer;
- Lymphoma;
- Leukemia;
- Cervical cancer;
- Ovarian cancer;
- Lung cancer.

Very often people (especially in the media, it seems) think Parkinson's is an old bloke's disease. Sadly, like the song says, it ain't necessarily so. It doesn't always hit after you turn 65, or even 60. About 18% of Australians diagnosed with PD are of working age, although many of them aren't working any more.

A part of the problem is that for most people the symptoms take years to develop and they live for a long time with the disease without even knowing it. Sometimes the symptoms aren't noticed. Sometimes they're noticed but not paid attention to. Sometimes they're noticed and recognised, but for various reasons the person with the disease doesn't want to admit it, to themselves or anyone else. And *that* is really a problem, because the longer it goes untreated the worse the symptoms will get.

> **Simply put:** if you suspect you've got a problem that might be Parkinson's, don't wait. Talk to your doctor.

Unlike some of the diseases that afflict people now PD is not a 21st century illness, or even a 20th century one. There are records of it going back to 5000 BC. Around that time, an ancient Indian civilization called the disorder *Kampavata*[2] (*kampa* is the Sanskrit word for 'tremor') and treated it with the seeds of a very particular plant. Those seeds contain a substance now called levodopa. It's the basis of the drug most commonly used in treating PD these days, and those seeds contain enough of it to be effective. The moral of that story: don't underestimate the 'old remedies'!

There are references to the disease, or something very like it, in ancient Chinese texts. And the Greek physician Galen, probably the first great student of anatomy, described what he called "shaking palsy" in 175AD.

That same term: "shaking palsy", was used by a London doctor named James Parkinson in a detailed medical essay published in 1817. He studied and reported on six cases of the condition among his own patients.

Sixty years later a French neurologist named Jean Martin Charcot did some serious follow-up work based on that essay. Charcot and his students studied and described the two main types of symptoms - tremors and rigidity. The Frenchman also recognised the London doctor's work by coining the name we now know: 'Parkinson's Disease'.

> **Simply put:** Parkinson's is really a
> disease affecting the chemistry of the brain,
> but we see the effects in the body.
> And it's been around for a very long time!

*

What Causes PD?

That, my friends, is a million-dollar question. Having taken about seven thousand years to figure out what Parkinson's Disease actually *is* (as distinct from just describing the symptoms), perhaps it's no surprise that nobody seems quite sure of exactly why those brain cells stop producing enough dopamine in some people but not others.

For a long time everyone seemed fairly sure that it's not **genetic**. There have been far too many cases of the disease hitting someone with no family history of it (or the reverse – two afflicted parents and no impact on the next generation/s) for anyone to think you're likely to be 'born with it'. Or without it.

But lately there's been some research that muddies the waters a bit. It seems that rather than a genetic *cause* for the disease, there may be something that makes some people more *likely* to get it.

It's a bit like lung cancer. Some people can smoke a pack a day for fifty years without getting lung cancer, while someone else seemingly just has to sit in a bus smelling of cigarette smoke a few times before they're diagnosed with it. (Seriously – a girl I grew up with died in her 20's in exactly those circumstances!) It's called a *genetic predisposition* to something. It doesn't mean you definitely *will* get whatever disease, just that the odds are tilted more against you.

In the case of PD, this genetic 'marker' isn't easy to spot. As one researcher put it:

> (it) may be subtle and difficult to detect in the absence of elaborate immunohistochemical techniques that, it is hoped, will become more widely applicable and available.[3]

What he means is that, like a lot to do with Parkinson's, the body chemistry happens at a very very microscopic level deep inside the brain, and is very very difficult to observe. But researchers and doctors are gradually getting better at knowing what to look for and where to look for it.

Simply put: A family history of Parkinson's Disease doesn't guarantee you'll get it, but it might make it more likely.

So if it's not genetic, what *is* the cause? Probably a combination of factors.

Age is usually regarded as one of them. But even that is misleading. PD gets recognised (i.e. diagnosed) more often in people over 60, but that might be because the symptoms tend to get worse over time. The early signs of the disease can easily be misdiagnosed or even overlooked – including by the sufferer, for as long as it takes until the symptoms are too obvious to miss or ignore.

There's no doubt that body chemistry changes with age, especially after menopause. Change of life, the 48 crash, mid-life crisis, whatever you want to call it. And yes, it does happen to men too. (Check out my book *Mid-life Crisis MANagement* for more information.) As the cocktail of chemicals in your body changes it's very likely that among the ones that suffers is dopamine.

One detailed study of nearly 600 PD patients found that 90% of them were diagnosed at the age of 50 or older.[4] That statistic seems pretty consistent in studies from around the world. (But remember: Statistics is the only science that enables different experts using the same figure to draw different conclusions.)

There is a positive side to the raw numbers. Once it *has* been diagnosed, the rate of the disease's progression is usually much slower in younger than older people.

That may well be due in part to the fact that younger people have fewer general health problems to make the problem worse, although I reckon that's less true than it used to be. Because they don't have as many other issues to contend with, younger sufferers are more capable of doing various physical therapy treatments that can reduce or slow down the effects of PD.

Simply put: age is a factor in two ways:
most people's bodies do gradually wear out
over time, and Parkinson's Disease is one of the
ways that 'wearing out' becomes apparent;
and because PD tends to progress slowly
many people aren't diagnosed until they're older
and their symptoms more severe.

There may be **environmental** factors that can trigger Parkinson's in someone who's got the body chemistry to make them vulnerable.

Chemical poisons like certain insecticides, fungicides and herbicides are possible causes of PD in some people. It's not universal, obviously. Some people use toxins at work every day for years with no ill effect. And not every PD sufferer has been exposed to such chemicals.

But there have been enough instances to suggest that there is a link. And enough evidence for the US Department of Veterans Affairs to officially recognize that exposure to Agent Orange is a significant contributor to the incidence of Parkinson's among service personnel.[5]

In case you missed it, or have forgotten, Agent Orange is a synthetic chemical herbicide. More than 20 million gallons of it were sprayed on vegetation and trees during the Vietnam War. The idea was to kill off the stuff that the enemy hid under, and the crops that they relied on for food. Trouble is that dioxin (one of the chemicals in the herbicide mix) is highly toxic even in minute amounts, and it affected the blokes preparing, transporting and spraying it as well as the *intended* victims.

Another environmental factor that has been suggested as having some influence in some cases of PD is exposure to metals and chemicals used in factories, such as manganese, lead, and trichlorethylene (TCE). And 'exposure' doesn't just mean at work in those factories – some of these things have a way of turning up in our water and food. Keep an eye and an ear out for reports in your local media about contamination, and don't dismiss them if they appear. Don't ignore a possibility of being poisoned.

Something else that's thought to increase the chances of getting Parkinson's is **head trauma**. Exactly how the link works isn't clear, but statistics and anecdotal evidence point to it as a potential factor.

There was an English study of PD in twins that found that where one twin was affected and the other wasn't, the affected twin was more likely to have sustained some sort of head trauma, even a mild one.[6]

Probably the best known example is Muhammad Ali, but he's certainly not the only ex-boxer, wrestler, footballer etc. to be diagnosed with PD in later life.

America's National Football League have established a program called the NFL Concussion Settlement to pay compensation to players (and especially ex-players) who've sustained head injuries that affect them later in life. It was assumed they'd mostly get claims about Alzheimers and dementia. There have been plenty of them, but also 107 claims relating to Parkinson's Disease in the first year. The NFL had expected fourteen. They'd expected to pay out about $7 million, but in the first year the figure was $47,071,554 – with a lot more cases to be finalised.[7]

The latest research I've seen – a study of over 160,000 people on the US

Veterans Health Administration database – looked at the correlation of 'traumatic brain injury' (TBI) and Parkinson's. It was found that those who'd had a "mild" TBI (a blow to the head with little or no loss of consciousness) had a 56% increased risk of developing PD. For those who'd had "moderate to severe" TBI (knocked out, extended unconsciousness, other long-term symptoms) that risk increased by a whopping 83%. There's some evidence that head injuries lead to deposits of 'abnormal proteins' in the brain, and that PD sufferers have been found to have an accumulation of these.[8]

I'm quite sure there'll be more debate about this. That seems to be the nature of studies in medicine, or science in general really, but I reckon there's enough to suggest that while a whack to the head might not be *the* cause of Parkinson's, there's a good chance that one or more of them is a significant part of what can trigger it.

Another possibility that's getting some attention is that PD has its origins not in the brain, but in **the gut**. This has come from studies in Denmark and Sweden. The researchers looked at people who'd had an operation called a *vagotomy*. That means the severing of the vagus nerve, a heavy-duty link that carries information (and microscopic body chemicals) back and forward between the intestine and the brain. Since the 1970's it's been done as a treatment for ulcers.

What they found is that people who'd had this link cut were statistically less likely to develop PD. In Sweden 19 people out of 9430 who'd had a complete vagotomy developed PD within five years – that's 0.78%. Compared to that 1.15% (3932 of 377,200) of people who didn't have the operation developed the disease in that same timeframe.[9]

The Danish study of 15,000 showed an even bigger difference. They found that patients who'd undergone a complete vagotomy were somehow 'protected' - their risk of developing PD over 20 years was half that of people whose vagus nerve was intact.[10]

Now, *why* this should be so is very much an open question. Both research teams made similar observations:

"Patients with Parkinson's disease are often constipated many years before they receive the diagnosis"[11] and "people with Parkinson's disease often have gastrointestinal problems such as constipation, that can start decades before they develop the disease."[12] That may or may not be a coincidence. Nobody has proposed a definite answer to explain the apparent connection. There are some theories, but until someone produces actual evidence of how it might work we can only include 'gastrointestinal problems' as one of PD's possible causes, or at least contributing factors.

Simply put: there doesn't seem to be any single cause for PD, but a combination of one or more environmental or physical things can trigger the disease.

.o0o.

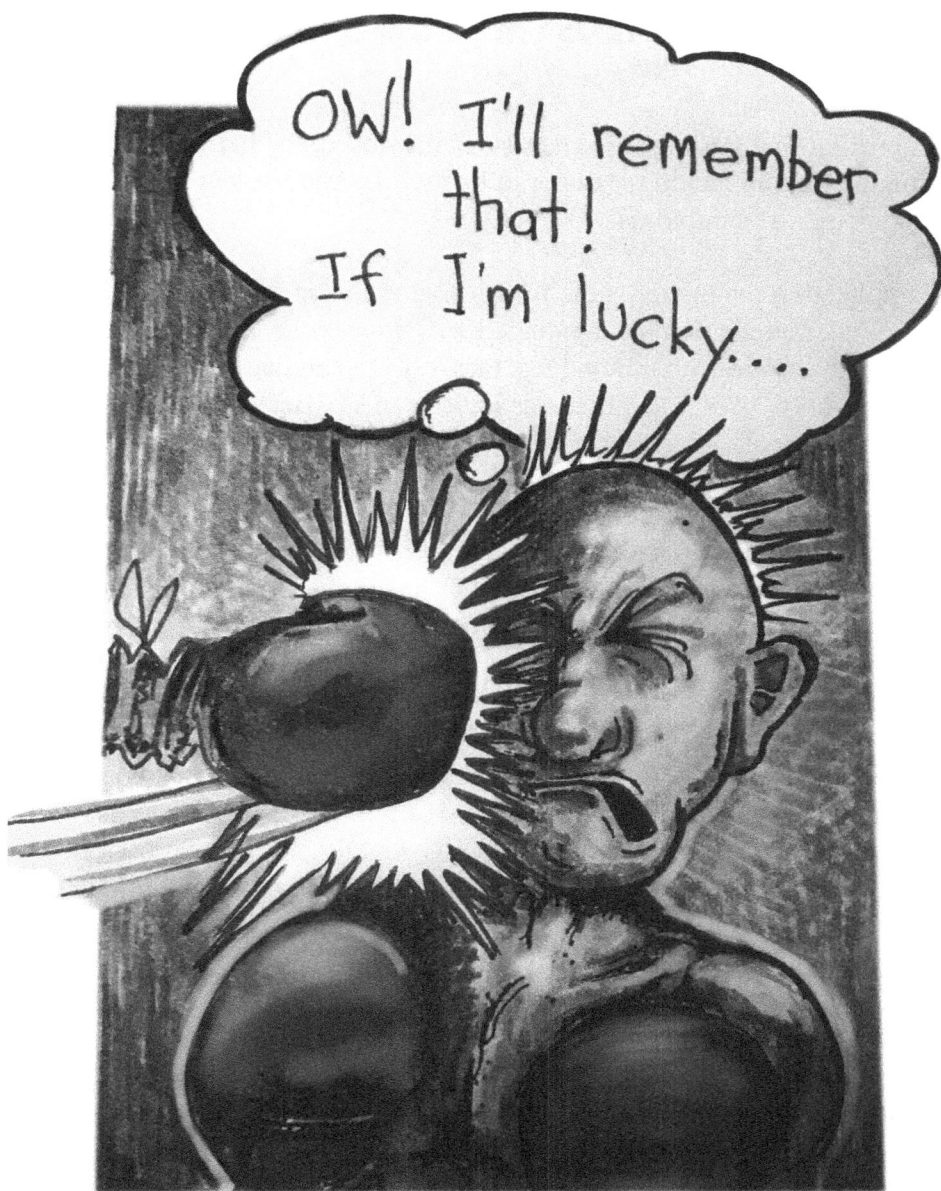

Head trauma might be one of the triggers of PD (pg 14)

2 WHAT ARE THE SYMPTOMS OF PD?

The earlier that Parkinson's Disease is diagnosed, the better the prospects of treating it and making it easier to live with. And the key to diagnosis is recognising the symptoms.

Complicating the matter is the fact that as yet there is no definitive test for PD. Well, there is, but it's conducted *post mortem* i.e. after you're dead. Prior to that there isn't a blood test or x-ray or scan that can tell a doctor with certainty, "Yes, this bloke has Parkinson's." Because there is no such test, and there are a number of other conditions that can produce similar symptoms (so much so that some are called 'parkinsonian conditions') there is a risk of misdiagnosis.

There is a new thing in the US called DaTscan that is an imaging technique that captures pictures of the dopamine system in the brain. It's pretty promising, but on its own it's not enough. DaTscan is really a means of confirming a clinical diagnosis based on a patient's symptoms.

For some people the progress of the disease and its symptoms is quicker and more obvious than for others. It's worth noting that for many, by the time the symptoms are severe enough to be really concerning, 60% to 80% of those dopamine-producing cells in the brain that I mentioned right at the start have stopped working. So it's really important to be aware of what's going on in your body.

The symptoms fall into two categories: 'motor' and 'non-motor'.

Motor symptoms are the best-known ones (especially for people who aren't in the medical profession). Broadly they involve some loss of voluntary movement and/or the presence of *in*voluntary movement. Often, but not always, they start on one side of the body, slowly getting worse and spreading to the other side.

Not everyone gets all of the same symptoms, and there can be a lot of variation in how severe they can get.

Tremors. Trembling in any or all of the fingers/hands/arms, the feet/ legs, even the head and jaw. Usually the tremors are more noticeable when the sufferer is resting rather than busy doing something. They may get worse when the person is excited, tired or stressed.

Rigidity. This particularly refers to stiffness of the limbs and trunk, which can actually get worse during movement. Often it produces aches and pains in the muscles. Rigidity can cause difficulty in tasks like writing, and even eating and drinking when it's hard to get your hand to your mouth!

Bradykinesia. It's the medical term for 'slowness of voluntary movement'. Not quite the same as 'rigidity', it often means difficulty in starting or completing movement. It can affect the facial muscles so the person looks like they're wearing an expressionless mask.

Impaired gait. Some PD sufferers walk with a distinctive shuffle, with shoulders stooped and their arms swinging less than normal (or not at all). It can be hard to make the first step, and to turn. Occasionally someone might 'freeze' in mid-stride and be at risk of falling forward.

Postural instability. Your balance as you walk and move around actually depends on constant adjustments to your posture: little bends left and right, forward and back. A lot of that happens without you being conscious of it. PD can get in the way of those little reflex movements, increasing the risk of falls.

Balance is a more complex business than you might realise. There's a thing called 'muscle sense' (or *proprioception*) that happens without your normally being aware of it (like breathing). Your body senses things like muscle length and tension, the position of joints, even the speed at which muscles extend and contract. That unconscious awareness feeds into what's called *kinaesthesia* – which is your conscious awareness of what your body is doing, how it's positioned and moving.

It seems like this proprioception may often be one of the first things impaired by PD. So you might, for instance, be taking shorter steps than you actually realise, and be more at risk of a fall. If someone with this problem starts to overbalance, they'll shift their feet to try to brace themselves, but not as far as they think they've done, and probably fall anyway.

These motor symptoms are the best-known signs of Parkinson's for most people. As a consequence of that, they're often the key to PD being diagnosed.

But it's by no means certain that they're actually the first symptoms of the disease to strike someone.

There are quite a number of **non-motor symptoms** that get ascribed to PD. Some relate to the changes in muscle control, while some seem to be linked to other aspects of the change in brain chemistry.

Speech difficulties. The voice becomes quieter and slower, and can sound monotone and expressionless.

Bladder problems. The need to pee can hit more often, and more urgently than it used to. There might also be incontinence issues, during day or night.

Constipation. On the other side of the coin, some of the muscles that move poop along your digestive system (and out of it) may be affected.

Erectile dysfunction. It becomes more difficult to get, or maintain, an erection. There's a depressingly long list of things that can cause this problem, but although it's not the most likely candidate, PD is certainly one of them.

Mouth problems. Swallowing might become difficult. Things might not taste the way they used to, although that may have as much to do with a diminished sense of smell as any effects on the taste buds on your tongue. And you might find you're producing more saliva, so you're swallowing more or spitting more. At its worst, that's how drooling comes about.

Excessive perspiration. Sweating more than you used to, and for less apparent reason ("I never used to raise a sweat walking to the corner store!").

Orthostatic hypotension. If your doctor tells you that you've got this, what it means is that your blood pressure is low when you're standing up. That can mean you're more at risk of being unsteady on your feet, or even falling over.

Mental problems. Things like confusion, memory loss and even dementia are sometimes associated with Parkinson's, particularly in elderly people. There's debate about whether they're directly connected, or coincidental as part of an overall pattern of age-related deterioration.

Mood disorders. Depression and anxiety can afflict a lot of PD patients. That makes a lot of sense – as you find yourself losing the mobility you used to enjoy it's natural to be upset or distressed about it. But it's potentially made worse by the chemical changes in your brain. Dopamine is important in helping you to feel pleasure (it's a 'reward signal' that tells your brain you've just got something you wanted) so when it doesn't get produced like it used to, you lose some of the sense of enjoyment of things.

REM behaviour disorder. Rapid eye movement behaviour disorder (RBD) is a sleep disorder that occurs during the REM sleep cycle – that is, when you're really deeply asleep. Normally a person doesn't move much when they're really deeply asleep. Apart from their eyes, the muscle tone relaxes. Someone with RBD moves as they sleep, especially their limbs. So much so it can seem like they're acting out their dreams, although that may not be the case – the movements might be random. The disorder is generally rare, but as many as 15% of people with PD may have RBD. It's not dangerous, but it's tiring because the body isn't getting a real rest. And it's no fun for anyone sharing the bed!

Other sleeping problems. With or without RBD complicating the matter, there may be other difficulties brought about by PD. Muscle activity, voluntary or otherwise, is tiring, so even if you're not particularly noticing the little 'extra' movements you may find you're sleeping too much during the day. Likewise, you may be sleeping too little at night without realising it's muscle discomfort or movement that's keeping you awake.

There are a lot of things that can contribute to any or all of these symptoms (both motor and non-motor) besides Parkinson's, but they're all 'warning flags'. If you're starting to notice any of them, then *listen to your body* – it's trying to tell you something!

Particularly if you do have a family history of PD, or if you know you've had one or more significant head knocks in the past, or you've been exposed to toxic chemicals. None of these things guarantee you've got, or will get Parkinson's – but when symptoms and known risk factors combine it makes sense to talk to a doctor or health professional, and look at taking action.

Remember: the doctor's job is to listen to you. One of the senior blokes at the Mayo Clinic wrote:

> "One thing I recognized early in my practice was the importance of listening to the people I was treating. They have taught me countless and invaluable lessons about PD that cannot be found in medical textbooks."[13]

If you feel like the person you're talking to isn't really listening, or worse – not taking you seriously – it's time to look for a second opinion. You should understand what they say to you, too. Hopefully this book will help, but don't be afraid to ask questions until you *do* understand. It's your body, and your life.

Simply put: PD has a list of potential symptoms, many but not all of them muscular. Be aware of changes in your body and take action before they get worse.

---

3 WHAT ARE THE STAGES OF PD?

Parkinson's Disease is a progressive degenerative disorder. That means as more cells in the brain break down, the symptoms – whatever they are in an individual case – get gradually worse.

Doctors (and even more typically, researchers) seem to delight in breaking progressive diseases and disorders down into 'Stages'. It can help refine diagnosis, and it's useful in case histories. If Dr. Smith reads a report from Dr. Lee that says a patient has "Stage 3 Parkinson's" then he/she has a better idea of the person's condition than if it just said that they "had PD".

Of course, it doesn't help that not everyone uses the same scale. Some list three stages, others list five, and there are some variations in the definitions of particular stages. They do at least all start at 1 for mild, and work up from there!

This is the list of stages used by the Parkinson's Foundation in the US. It's pretty simple and descriptive, and most of the others seem to be variations on the same basic theme.

Stage 1: Mild symptoms (tremors and/or movement symptoms like swinging arm while walking) that don't interfere with daily activities, and occur on one side of the body

Stage 2: Symptoms worsen with walking problems and both sides of the body are affected. Some secondary symptoms may be noticed

Stage 3: Main symptoms worsen with loss of balance and slowness of movement

Stage 4: Severity of symptoms means that help is regularly required; usually the person cannot live alone

Stage 5: A care provider is needed for all activities. The patient may not be able to stand or walk unaided, and may be bedridden. They may also have hallucinations and/or delusions.[14]

There's no hard-and-fast rule about how long it takes to go from any one stage to the next. It's different for every patient. Nor is it predictable – someone might go from Stage 1 to Stage 2 quite quickly, then remain at that level for many years without degenerating into Stage 3 or beyond.

Your own personal 'history' is what's most important in the diagnosis. If you, or someone close to you, notice changes in your movements and/or speech, then mention it to your doctor, sooner rather than later. No matter how vague or even silly the doctor's questions might seem, be as honest and direct in your answers as you possibly can. Don't try to guess at a 'right' answer, just give an honest one.

Often, especially in the early stages, the suggestion might be to "wait and see". That's okay. It shouldn't actually mean "do nothing" - this is the time for the doctor (and you!) to start paying attention and making some notes. What are you noticing? What things are getting harder to do? How much harder, and in what way?

Does your hand shake when you pick up a cup of coffee or a beer? Which hand? All the time, or only when you're tired? Maybe you've noticed a problem with stairs. Going up, or down, or both? Is it worse on the left or right foot?

Simple as those sound, they're important. If you establish some bench-marks early, you and the doctor both have a much better chance of actually recognising deterioration as it happens. It doesn't always happen quickly, and sometimes the slowness means that Parkinson's 'sneaks up' on some-one.

Everyone seems to have their own natural 'rate of decay' of those import-ant brain cells based on their own body chemistry. Furthermore it seems that many of the questions around what **causes** Parkinson's also apply to how quickly or slowly it progresses. There are things that might make matters worse, but there are also things that can help slow down the dete-rioration. Some of them are things that you can do for yourself. Others require some professional help.

That unpredictability is really a positive thing. The rate of progression of PD isn't 'locked in'. The earlier it can be recognised (or admitted to!), the sooner steps can be taken to do something about slowing the progress of the disease. I'll spend the second half of this book examining different things that might help to achieve that.

> **Simply put:** The symptoms of PD get worse gradually. The earlier you recognise and start doing something about them, the more you can slow the rate of decline.

.o0o.

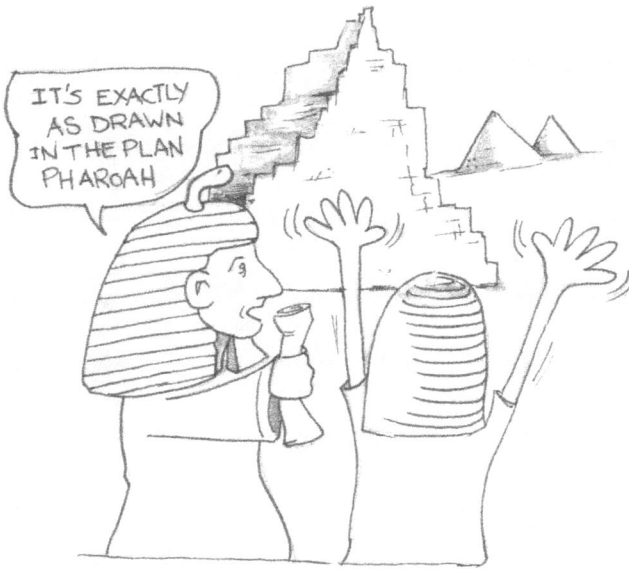

It seems the Royal Architect has a problem...

Parkinson's Disease has been around for a VERY
long time (pg 10)

4 WHAT'S DIFFERENT FOR MEN?

It doesn't seem fair (nothing much about Parkinson's Disease seems fair) but blokes are at least one-and-a-half times more likely to get PD than women. A large study by the American Journal of Epidemiology pushed that out to almost a two to one margin.[15]

The obvious question is "why?" Unfortunately, to answer it with any certainty we'd have to know a lot more about the real causes of the disease. There are a few things that do seem to contribute though.

One of them is to do with body chemistry, in particular the hormone *oestrogen*. Usually thought of as **the** primary female sex hormone, it's worth noting that males naturally produce it too – just not in the same quantity.

There was a study published in the *Journal of Neurology, Neurosurgery & Psychiatry* that found that a woman who experiences later menopause, or has more children, is more likely to have delayed onset of PD symptoms. Both of these things tend to indicate she has a higher than average level of oestrogen in her body.[16]

So there's an implied link between oestrogen and the cells that produce dopamine. The suggestion is that the hormone works to protect the brain cells (it's called a 'neuroprotectant'). Higher levels of oestrogen can apparently mean that the gradual breakdown that is PD starts later – or not at all – and happens more slowly.

There are some other differences between men and women that may contribute to the imbalance in the statistics. Not so much physical things, but different circumstances that relate to some of the potential causes of Parkinson's. It's a matter of statistics.

Things are changing, but I reckon over past decades there have been more men than women working in occupations that expose them to the various toxic chemicals and materials implicated in PD.

And then there's the matter of head trauma. Accidents can happen to any-body, but a lot of head trauma is sports-related, particularly contact sports. Think of the injuries, big and small sustained in football (whatever code).

Players landing on their head after taking a great mark in Aussie Rules; the impact of an arm or the ground during a heavy tackle in one of the rugby codes; innumerable small blows to the skull heading a soccer ball; every tackle in a gridiron game rattles the brain against bone in a way that no helmet can prevent. Then there's boxing and professional wrestling, where participants make their living from being hit in the melon.

It's only in recent years that women have been participating in these sports in significant numbers. Give it several years, but I reckon that, in time, we might start to see the number of women suffering from PD increase.

Parkinson's doesn't just distinguish between the sexes on the raw num-bers of who's afflicted. There are also distinctions in symptoms – what and even when they strike. The average age of diagnosis for women is two years later than for men.

There's no hard rule, but the first major motor symptom in women is often tremor (67%, as compared to 48% of male PD sufferers[17]) whereas men more commonly start with that slow or rigid movement called *bradykine-sia*. The 'tremor-type' PD is associated with a slower disease progression and generally a better quality of life than the 'bradykinesia' type, and yet "women often report less satisfaction with their quality of life, even with a similar level of symptoms" according to one (female) researcher.[18]

When bradykinesia affects the muscles of the face it can 'freeze' into something like a mask. So PD patients can have trouble showing emotion facially. Maybe somehow because of that, or maybe coincidentally, they can also begin to have difficulty interpreting others' expressions. One study suggests that although both men and women with PD can have diffi-culty interpreting anger and surprise, it seems that men are more likely to lose the ability to interpret fear.

The effects of Parkinson's go beyond the physical, and there's some evidence those effects also differ according to gender. For instance, men appear to retain a better ability to understand spatial orientation – a better sense of where they are and how to move around their environment safely. Women, on the other hand, retain more verbal fluency, so their speech is easier to understand.

I referred earlier to Rapid eye movement Behaviour Disorder (RBD) affecting the muscle activity of as many as 15% of PD sufferers while they sleep. According to the journal *International Review of Psychiatry* men are much more likely to have this condition than women.[19]

Finally, the psychological reaction to Parkinson's seems to be different for blokes. It's suggested that women with PD tend to experience a higher rate of depression than men with PD do. A key part of the 'evidence' for this is that women sufferers are recorded as being prescribed antidepressant medication more often.

Let's recognise though that we blokes aren't as good as women at admitting to depression – even to ourselves far less anyone else like a doctor. It doesn't mean we're less likely to suffer from it, just less likely to appear on the medical statistics.

What do show up on those statistics are things that are often outside a sufferer's control. Things like wandering, or even uncharacteristic anti-social behaviour – the sort of inappropriate or abusive behaviour that gets treated by antipsychotic medications. Records do get kept about such things, and they suggest that men are more likely to fall into this category than women.

I haven't seen any evidence, or even suggestion that PD, for all that it's a brain disorder, has a direct chemical or physical link to anti-social behaviour. But it does seem very much as though more women get depressed about their deteriorating condition, while more blokes get aggressive about it. They're simply two different responses to the experience of living with PD.

Neither does there seem to be any suggestion that any particular treatment is more or less useful for either gender. Even if the link between oestrogen and PD is conclusively proven, there's no reason that some sort of hormone therapy would only work for one sex. Oestrogen does naturally occur in both men and women, after all.

Simply put: men seem more likely to get Parkinson's than women. They may have different symptoms, and they may react differently to the effects. The treatments available are the same for everyone though.

.o0o.

5 WHAT THERAPIES MIGHT HELP?

At the moment, Parkinson's may be a life sentence but it's not a **death** sentence. And it's important to remember that there are things that you can do to improve the quality of that life.

These are not 'cures'. So far there isn't one, although a lot of time and money is going into looking for one. They're ways of relieving symptoms – even slowing down or reversing the steady decline that is PD. But a 'cure' relies on knowing a 'cause'. The search goes on.

There is no one thing that's guaranteed to succeed in helping you to overcome or even live with Parkinson's. But there is one thing that is guaranteed to fail, and that one thing is doing nothing.

While doctors and scientists and patients and carers continue to search for answers, a range of options is available which can, in different ways, help. They may slow the rate of deterioration caused by the disease, they may reduce or control particular symptoms, or they may make the condition easier to cope with.

Some work on the body, some work on the brain. And some work on the mind, which is not necessarily the same thing.

I can't stress enough: there is no 'one size fits all' solution. What works for one person isn't guaranteed to work for another.

But no therapy has a chance of helping if you're not willing to give it a go. A **genuine** go – not a half-hearted 'going through the motions' pretence at an effort. I know it's become a cliché to say, "You get out what you put in", but clichés often start out by simply being true.

It might mean the self-discipline to remember to take a particular medication every day at the same time. It might mean the persistence to haul yourself off to an exercise class, or some other regular activity, even when the weather's lousy or you're tired or there's a good match on the telly.

It might even mean trying something new! Some blokes love a challenge like that, but I know there are plenty who aren't so keen.

Your choice, really. Be willing to show some commitment and give something a go, or be prepared to steadily lose control of your body and ultimately your life.

> **Simply put:** there is only one way to know
> if a treatment is effective for you,
> and that's to really try it.

*

5.1 Drugs

At present there's one medication that's prescribed far more often than any other. It's called *levodopa*. It's a naturally occurring substance that was used seven thousand years ago in India to treat what we now call Parkinson's Disease.

It actually converts to dopamine inside the brain. It doesn't replace what's already been lost but effectively reduces the rate of deterioration, so slows down the symptoms. Unfortunately prolonged use of levodopa has unpleasant side effects such as painful cramps and involuntary movements. Furthermore, with each dose the response time – the time for which the drug is effective - gets shorter. Because of this its prescription is often delayed until the disease is in its later stages and the symptoms are more severe.

In another one of those curious differences between the genders levodopa is metabolized differently in men compared to women. That may be something to do with men generally having a larger body mass, so the dosage for men with PD is usually higher than for women. And it's women who are more likely to suffer badly from the drug's side effects.[20]

To deal with some of those side-effects levodopa is often prescribed together with another drug – *carbidopa*. This drug protects the levodopa from being broken down and absorbed by other parts of the body before it reaches the brain. By combining the two a lower dose of levodopa will produce the same benefit with less side effects.[21]

By the way, it seems that broad beans are a good natural source of levodopa. I've read that 100 grams of broad beans provides a dose of about 250mg of the stuff. Much of that is in the actual bean pod, so if you're trying it out, remember to eat the pods too.

Not everyone is helped by levodopa. It's been suggested that maybe five to ten percent of PD sufferers fail to respond to the drug[22]. In such cases, as well as instances when levodopa has been taken long enough to reduce its effectiveness below a valuable threshold, or when the side effects are too severe to be persisted with, a variety of other drugs may be prescribed. These target symptoms in various ways, such as suppressing muscle or nerve activity.

The big danger is that these drugs also come with their own side effects. These become more drastic and less predictable when different drugs are combined. Some of these 'cocktails' don't just affect the body (notably the liver and kidneys) but can also do psychological damage. Reactions ranging from depression to aggression have been reported.

One example is *rapamycin*. It prevents the death of nerve cells in the brain, which sounds like a good thing for dopamine production. The trouble is that it suppresses the immune system (it's actually used in transplant patients to combat tissue rejection) and that opens up the prospect of a whole big raft of side effects for PD sufferers.

The other type of drug therapy that's used is a substance called a ***dopamine agonist***. An 'agonist' is a substance that acts like another substance in the body, and therefore stimulates the same action/reaction as what it duplicates. So a 'dopamine agonist' is a drug that produces the same effects as the dopamine the brain is no longer making enough of.

There are a few types of these available, usually administered by tablet, injection, or a 'patch' worn on the skin. One example is *apomorphine* (which, despite the name, has nothing to do with morphine). This is one of those administered by needle – either an injection, or infusion using a small pump. If it's prescribed for you then you should get full instructions on how and when to take it.

Agonists like apomorphine tend to be prescribed for patients in later stages of PD, when symptoms are no longer responding as well or as consistently to the likes of levodopa (although both drugs may be prescribed at the same time). And like levodopa, they don't work for everyone.

An important benefit of these drugs is that they can act as a 'rescue', like insulin for a diabetic. For someone whose symptoms sometimes 'kick in' suddenly this can be very valuable! Injections especially are fast-acting. Apomorphine takes effect within 5 to 10 minutes, much faster than tablets. It wears off within 40 minutes, but by then the regular oral medication should be working.

If a dopamine agonist treatment is used regularly over an extended period of months, some patients find the number of times that their symptoms 'flare up' is significantly reduced.

On the other hand, there are some negatives to such a treatment beyond the difficulty some patients have with trying to safely inject themselves.

As with any drug, there is a risk of side effects, some of which can be quite serious. The data sheet for apomorphine, for instance, lists the following possible impacts:

-   Nausea and vomiting (in which case another anti-nausea drug will be added to the prescription mix);

-   Drop in blood pressure;

-   Anaemia and other blood disorders (in rare cases);

-   Fainting or heart palpitations (especially in patients with existing heart conditions);

-   Drowsiness or sudden onset of sleep;

-   Skin reaction e.g. rash or nodules at or around the point of injection;

-   Hallucinations or delusions;

- Impulsive or compulsive behaviour e.g. gambling or 'binge' eating.

There was also some research around 2001 that suggested that both agonists and levodopa might worsen a patient's proprioception (muscle sense), so things like balance may actually get a bit worse. I've since been told by a very respected authority that more recent studies haven't supported that earlier interpretation, and that dopamine replacement therapy actually restores muscle sense by about 20-30% in patients with mild to moderate PD.[23]

I've just read some very new research out of the University of Queensland Institute for Molecular Bioscience that examines a substance called NLRP3 inflammasome, which is highly activated in PD sufferers. It's closely related to the deterioration in those dopamine-producing brain cells. The research team found that a small molecule (MCC950) effectively 'cooled down' inflammation and allowed the relevant cells to function normally.

What that meant was that there was a measurable decrease in the development of PD in the test subjects – not just symptoms, but the disease itself. The catch is that those test subjects were mice.

One of the research team, Professor Matt Cooper, said that they were looking forward to progressing their research through to clinical trials using the MCC950 molecule in oral drug form. He hopes that, depending on funding, those trials might commence in 2020.[24]

As with any treatment, responses to medication will vary from person to person. What drug is prescribed, what dose, and the timing might, perhaps *should* vary between patients according to things like what stage the disease is at, what other medications they're on, and their own health history. Drug therapy should be individualized, and the results monitored right from the start.

Nobody knows your own body and mind better than you do. If you notice changes in your physical condition, mood or behaviour after starting a new course of medicines, **tell** the person who prescribed them. That said, if people around you start telling you, "Jeez mate, you've changed!" (and they don't mean it in a good way) listen to them. And again, talk to whoever put you on the new drug/s. Between you and the doctor you can decide whether the good effects of the medication outweigh the negatives. Remember, it's your life, and should be *your* decision either way.

Simply put: there are no drugs to "cure" PD.
Some can relieve symptoms, but you should
be aware of any side effects and talk
to your doctor about them.

---

*

5.2 Surgery - DBS

When drugs aren't effective it's not unusual for 'Western medicine' to turn to the scalpel for means of relief, if not cure. It's no different in the treatment of Parkinson's.

Until fairly recently there were two surgical options – *pallidotomy* and *thalamotomy*. Both of these involved surgically destroying or interfering with parts of the brain responsible for particular symptoms. Risky, difficult, and focused on effects, not causes. They were never common, and are getting even less so.

In their place as a surgical option now is a procedure called ***deep brain stimulation (DBS)***. This involves placing electrodes in specific areas of the brain of a PD sufferer. The electrodes are connected to a generator, which is programmed to send electrical impulses to decrease symptoms by interrupting the 'wrong' signals that are going from the head to the body.

DBS has a number of limitations.
• It's pretty invasive surgery on the brain, which is inherently risky;
• If there are any other conditions/diseases going on its effectiveness can be a lot less;
• It works on some (not all) motor symptoms but not many others;
• It can cause memory or reasoning problems;

- The electrode can dislodge – not dangerous in itself, but it means more surgery to fix the problem.

Usually DBS becomes seriously considered when medication has stopped working effectively, or consistently, to control symptoms. The dosage might be getting too high for comfort, or the patient is having more 'off' periods when the drugs seem to have little or no impact.

A general rule is that DBS will probably improve Parkinson's symptoms that respond to medication. Unfortunately the opposite is also true: many symptoms that aren't getting better with medication probably won't respond to DBS.

One thing research shows is that DBS surgery is particularly good for improving proprioception. It seems that the direct stimulation to the brain enhances that 'muscle sense' that's crucial for safe balance.

For the right patients, DBS can be very good for lessening symptoms and medication requirements. By allowing lower dosage it can decrease the side effects that can accompany drug therapy. It also doesn't have the same negative effect on 'muscle sense' that drugs often do, and that's a good thing.

> **Simply put:** surgical options may treat some Parkinson's symptoms. They aren't a cure, and do have some potential risks.

*

5.3 Exercise

Pretty much *the* most important and helpful thing that someone with Parkinson's can do for their own benefit is exercise. I don't mean a bunch of star-jumps and push-ups, or a ten kilometre run every day (although either may work for some people). I mean deliberate, repetitive ***movement***, however small and gentle, that helps to build muscle control.

There are plenty of ways to do this, but the specialist therapist that a good doctor is most likely to refer you to is an ***exercise physiologist***.

The American Society of Exercise Physiologists definition of what they do includes:

- the identification of physiological mechanisms underlying physical activity,
- the comprehensive delivery of treatment services concerned with the analysis, improvement and maintenance of health and fitness,
- rehabilitation of... chronic diseases and/or disabilities.[25]

What that all boils down to is a person who is trained to understand how the body is supposed to move, and how to use the right movements as a way to deal with a range of physical problems.

It's a lot more than being a gym instructor with a fancy title. An exercise physiologist will talk to an individual and assess that person's own particular issues – muscle weakness, balance problems, or tremors for example. Then, based on that assessment they'll put together an exercise program to address those issues.

The program might include exercises targeting cardio, strength, balance, or the flexibility/function of one or more specific body parts. More likely it'll be a combination of a few of those.

It's likely that the program will gradually build in intensity. As the body gets stronger and is capable of doing more, it makes sense to keep challenging it.

As you progress through a planned program, two things are happening: the muscles themselves get stronger with regular use, and the control of movement gets better with practice. Neither of which will *cure* PD, but they certainly will make it easier to cope with many of the symptoms.

You get out what you put in. For best results, do your exercises regularly, and to the best of your ability.

38

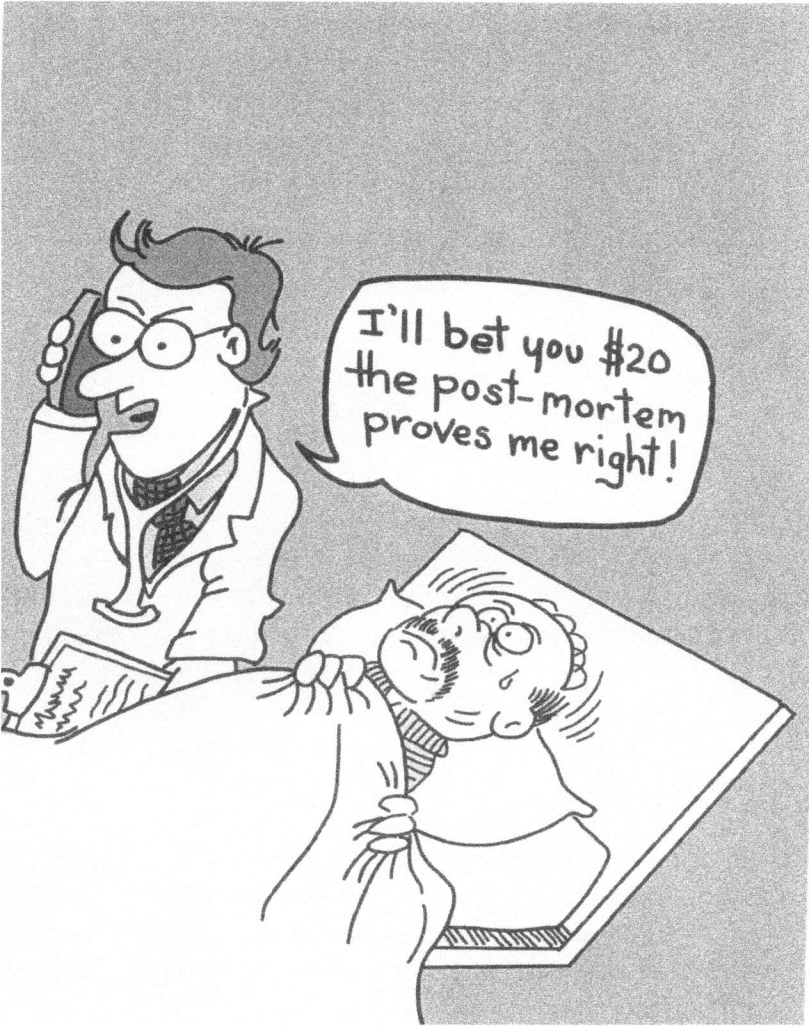

The only definitive test for Parkinson's Disease has to be conducted **post-mortem**. (pg 18)

> **Simply put:** Movement and exercise are
> extremely important and beneficial
> in dealing with the symptoms of PD.
> Specially targeted exercise can be
> especially helpful.

*

5.4 Physiotherapy and 'PD Warrior'

It seems like every professional sports team now has at least one physio-therapist on the staff. They've become the 'go-to' medical professionals for treating sports injuries, but also for dealing with the very real day-to-day aches and pains of everyone from accident victims to overworked gardeners.

On their website (www.physiotherapy.asn.au) the Australian Physiothera-py Association describe their members' role like this:

> Using advanced techniques and evidence-based care, physiother-apists assess, diagnose, treat and prevent a wide range of health conditions and movement disorders. Physiotherapy helps repair damage, reduce stiffness and pain, increase mobility and improve quality of life.

It's a natural fit for physiotherapists to be at the front line of helping PD patients. So much so that there are now very specific training courses for physios on managing Parkinson's patients.

If you choose to see a physio, or are referred to one, just ask whether he or she has had that additional training. It's not essential, but it would be helpful in their understanding of what you can and can't do.

Their work is closely aligned with what an exercise physiologist (EP) may do (see **5.3** above), but there are some differences. While an EP might be more inclined to look at a 'whole of life' program (including diet and other behaviour patterns) a physiotherapist could be a bit more 'hands on' in helping with exercises and manipulating some affected body parts.

In theory, a physiotherapist would usually deal with the acute phase of an injury or condition i.e. new pain, to relieve the initial problem. An EP then manages a longer term treatment to stabilize or even overcome the underlying condition. In reality, the line between the two is not that clear, especially when it comes to Parkinson's.

A really good example of this is the ***PD Warrior*** program. First developed by an Australian specialist physiotherapist named Melissa McConaghy, it's a comprehensive package that brings together exercise treatments, education, and a strong motivational support network specifically targeting not only the body, but the areas of the brain that are affected by Parkinson's.

Designed to slow down the effects of the condition, PD Warrior features exercises designed to train the brain to control the body better, and ultimately help patients move better and more confidently. Essentially, it gives patients confidence in their movement and therefore a better quality of life[26].

Again, it's not a 'quick fix', and qualified PD Warrior instructors will admit that it can be quite challenging, especially in the early stages. Some of the exercise movements can be quite exaggerated and feel awkward at first. The key is in the support and the education that allows participants to continue a safe home exercise program that's designed to 'reprogram' the brain. The brain has some natural ability to protect itself, and this therapy is intended to encourage that. The deterioration of 'muscle sense' that I mentioned in **Chapter 2** is something that may be particularly helped by the input of a good physiotherapist or exercise physiologist, as their programs can do a lot to improve body awareness.

So the physiotherapist's role is going beyond pain management. He or she is directly helping with mobility, stability, co-ordination and flexibility.

Key word there: helping. As with so many therapies, success depends on the person being treated putting in effort themselves and persisting with the program that's set for them.

Simply put: A suitably trained and qualified physiotherapist can help devise a program to improve some of the physical symptoms of PD, working with the active participation of the patient.

---

*

5.5 Traditional Chinese Medicine and Massage

Approaches to healing have evolved along quite different pathways in the 'West' and 'East'. Although it's been 'catching up' now, for many years 'Western' medicine has focused very much on the treatment of symptoms – how to ease the pain of that headache, unblock that constipation etc. Drugs and surgery have been used to target effects more often than underlying causes.

Traditional Chinese medicine (TCM) looks more closely at the interconnectedness of things. Mind, body and spirit are related directly to one another, as are various systems within the body. That's how a needle in the back of your hand can ease a pain in the kidney, or a particular herbal tea can be used to treat anger.

Because of this fundamental technique of looking more broadly at things, TCM offers a few approaches to Parkinson's Disease that aren't yet widely recognised in other cultures.

The holistic approach (i.e. different areas of the body are directly linked with each other on particular pathways) is central to Chinese healing. It's

42

what underpins acupuncture – more on that in the next section – but is also important in other techniques and therapies. For example I've read a very specific instruction to practitioners using reflexology massage:

'Walk the thumb over the area of the diaphragm and solar plexus to help with tremors associated with the disease, and work your way up the spinal column to help stabilize the nervous system.

Pressing the following points for a good three minutes each time can help with the symptoms to a considerable extent.

- Pituitary.

- Cerebrum.

- Cerebellum.

- Spine.

- Kidney.

- Adrenal.

- Liver.

- Autonomic nervous system.

Working on the reflexes of the entire spine can bring about alertness and confidence that ebbs away when the disease sets in.'[27]

(Bear in mind these 'points' are not necessarily on or near the organ they're named for. It'd be pretty difficult to press directly on the cerebellum, which is right inside your brain! The 'points' are on the 'pathways' that link the interconnected bits of the body's systems.)

As that indicates, TCM practitioners often have high regard for massage as a good therapy for PD patients. It makes sense for a condition marked by muscle stiffness and movement difficulty.

Massage is probably the oldest and most instinctive treatment for pain there is. Think about it – in every culture, in every part of the world, when someone is hurt their first reaction is to touch, or rub the sore spot – and it often does make it feel better! It's a reflex response to pain. So you can argue that massage is really our oldest therapy.

If you've ever had a good massage you'll know how much better and looser your muscles and joints can feel afterwards. That's a useful result for someone with Parkinson's – not only do they feel better, but they're also in a better condition to move themselves and get some more exercise. And I'll stress yet again: *exercise is the real key to dealing with PD*.

It doesn't matter if it's Chinese, Swedish, Thai, or Hawaiian, as long as it's good. And delivered by someone who is comfortable working on a client who has PD.

It *shouldn't* make any difference: every massage should be done with the pressure that the client wants. But some massage therapists (especially those whose training has been a bit rough and ready) won't know how to deal with someone for whom the wrong pressure in the wrong place could trigger a spasm or sudden burst of tremors. If you're going for a massage it's important you talk to the person working on you, both before and during the procedure.

One warning I must give around massage as a remedial therapy – for safety's sake you *must* be able to *feel* the area being worked on. If your shoulder/hip/knee or whatever is numb then it shouldn't be worked on. The person giving the massage can only judge how much pressure to apply based on your reactions. If you can't feel any sensation then neither you nor the therapist know if you're actually being damaged by what's being done.

Chinese medicine also sets great store by herbal remedies. Before you roll your eyes, wrinkle your nose and dismiss them, remember that some of these concoctions have been used, and working, for a very long time. And one that's particularly prescribed for PD has a good pedigree.

A herb called **gou teng** has been used by Chinese healers for over 2000 years to treat people with "the shakes". A 2011 trial of 115 Parkinson's patients clearly showed volunteers taking the herb slept better and spoke more fluently after thirteen weeks than those who'd been taking a 'placebo' preparation.[28]

Some serious research is now going into *why* this is the case. At **5.1** I mentioned a drug called *rapamycin* that protects against the destruction of brain cells. It seems that *gou teng* does a similar job, but does it without depressing the body's immune system. It's been taken for centuries without any such serious side effects being noted. Research in Hong Kong and Canada has identified a specific compound in *gou teng* (it's called *isorhy* if you're interested) that appears to be the 'active ingredient' that works rather like *rapamycin*, but along different pathways in the brain. Maybe that's why it doesn't have the same side effects.

The detailed research is a work in progress, but the evidence of centuries of experience seems pretty positive.

Simply put: Traditional Chinese healing offers
a range of ways of dealing with Parkinson's
based on many hundreds of years
of experience and practice.

---

*

5.6 Acupuncture

In the same way that massage therapy can offer relief from the symptoms of PD, so too can acupuncture.

Again, it's not a cure. But there's good evidence that acupuncture can significantly help to relieve some of the symptoms of Parkinson's. It works by interrupting some of the signals that flow through the body along both nerves and the 'pathways' that Chinese therapists call *qi* channels, or acupuncture channels. Similar to the pathways of the nervous system, these are described as 'lines' along which energy flows, connecting various parts of the body as I mentioned in **5.5** above. A needle or needles in the right point/s can block pain, or block the PD-affected signals from the brain that cause things like tremors. There are also now some therapists who'll use a laser instead of the traditional needles, but this isn't common yet.

There are two particular points that therapists target to treat some of the more common symptoms. They're called LV3 and GB34. I'm not going to explain exactly where they are because I don't want anyone to stick pins into themselves trying out DIY acupuncture. But just to give you some idea (so you have some appreciation of what a therapist may be doing) LV3 is on the top of the foot, and has historically been used to treat tremors (and a lot else). GB34 is on the outside of the leg below the knee and is traditionally associated with paralysis and painful tendon, ligament and joint disorders, as well as a variety of other conditions.[29]

I'll get technical for a minute to explain how it actually works. Scientists at the World Health Organization Collaborating Centre for Traditional Medicine have discovered that these two acupuncture points, as well as interfering with signals along energy channels, also prevent the breakdown of an important brain-protecting enzyme, tyrosine hydroxylase. This enzyme helps the body to create L-DOPA, an important dopamine precursor and drug used in the treatment of Parkinson's disease. It is now known that acupuncture prevents decreases of the L-DOPA creating enzyme in the thalamic portions of the brain thereby improving the motor function that is destroyed by Parkinson's[30].

What all that means is that targeting those two points LV3 and GB34 can apparently help to slow down the deterioration of brain cells that's the nub of PD.

A major study in 2015/16 across three countries looked at controlled trials of acupuncture as a treatment for Parkinson's, both as a 'stand-alone' and in combination with other 'conventional' Western treatments. The findings across twenty-five different trials were summarized:
    "Acupuncture was effective in relieving PD symptoms compared

with no treatment and conventional treatment alone, and acupuncture plus conventional treatment had a more significant effect than conventional treatment alone."[31]

Another potentially useful 'point' is HT7, which is on your wrist. A 2014 study in Thailand looked at laser acupuncture of the equivalent point in rats, and found a lot of positive results in reducing neuron degeneration and memory impairment, and improving dopamine production. By the researchers' own admission though, more research is required. What works on rats is a good guide, but not guaranteed to work on humans.

Not every acupuncturist is willing or able to try to treat Parkinson's. It's specialist work and they should have had appropriate training before they tackle it. That said, it's a therapy with runs on the board and so it may be worth your while to seek out someone with the right skill and experience.

There's a therapy called *electroacupuncture* or EA that takes the basic principle of acupuncture (applying needles to points on the energy channels) and ramps it up by adding electrical impulses through the needles.

I've read a study of a trial of fifty PD patients, half of whom were given a combination of drug and EA treatment while half got the drugs only. Those who received the electroacupuncture showed significant improvement in both motor symptoms (tremor, rigidity, bradykinesia) and non-motor symptoms such as depression and sleep disturbances. The results were particularly good for patients in the earlier stages of Parkinson's[32]. It's too small a study to be absolutely conclusive, but it's a good result, and certainly reinforces the positive research about acupuncture in general.

Scalp acupuncture is a similar therapy, but the needles are inserted on a different set of lines on the scalp to those of 'traditional' acupuncture. There are several studies out of China that indicate scalp acupuncture (including mild electroacupuncture), used in combination with other treatments such as levodopa, can significantly improve dopamine production and alleviate PD symptoms. Results were noticeably better over a three month study than those conducted over 30 days, which suggests that, as with many therapies, it's a good idea to be patient.

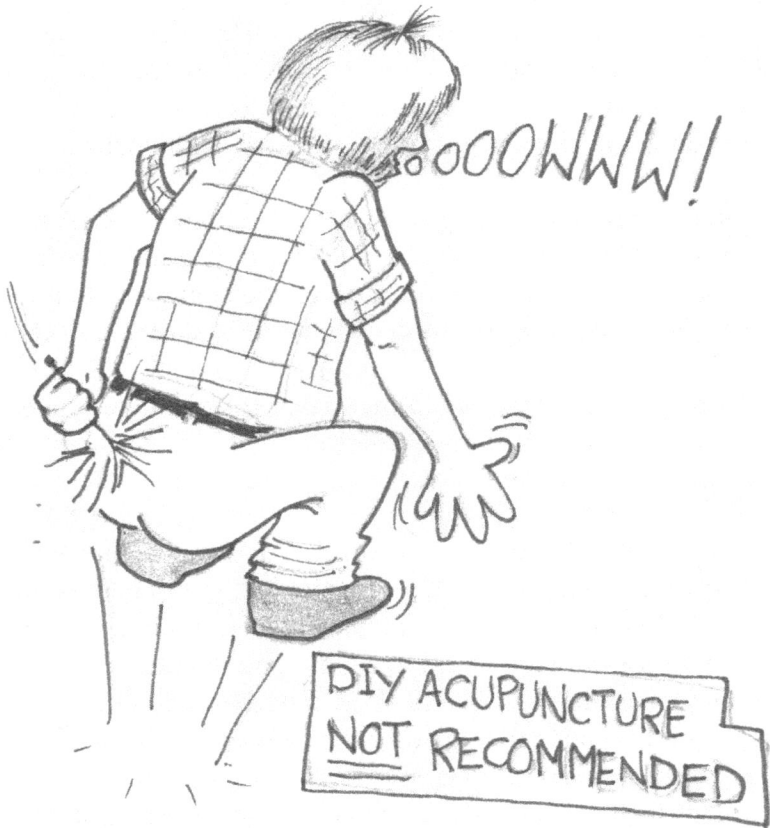

I'm **not** going to tell you exactly where to stick the needles. (pg 46)

Those Chinese studies were supported by a rigorous three month long study in Germany in 2015. It found an average of 38% improvement in mood, thinking and behaviour between the start and end of the trial, and an average 28% in daily activities affected by motor symptoms. There were only sixty people involved in the trial, but it's certainly encouraging.

> **Simply put:** Acupuncture can potentially disrupt some of the faulty 'signals' to the muscles associated with PD symptoms, offering relief from those symptoms.

*

5.7 Medical cannabis

One of the most controversial options put out there for Parkinson's patients is the therapeutic use of marijuana. I find that a bit strange, because the stuff's been being used for medicinal purposes across the world for thousands of years. It was a prescribed botanical medicine in the 19th and early 20th centuries.

Yes, I know it has a lot of potential to be a 'drug of addiction'. So do many painkillers, not to mention alcohol, tobacco and caffeine. Yes, it has side effects. So do many painkillers, not to mention alcohol, tobacco and caffeine.

In an uncontrolled market there is certainly some dodgy stuff out there. Impure, contaminated, past its best – there are plenty of potential problems.

But grown under good conditions, especially free of chemical fertilizers and pesticides etc., a medicinal grade cannabis plant can produce something that's very effective.

The key therapeutic bit of cannabis is ***cannabidiol***.

Technical time again. Skip ahead if chemistry isn't your thing, but I'll try to make it as clear as I can. In your body is a thing called the *endocannabinoid system* or ECS. It's one of a number of systems of neurotransmitters (like dopamine) that move signals from one part of your body to another. Inside the brain it's connected with areas associated with motor control, as well as a range of other functions like reproduction and sleep. Cannabidiol reacts with the ECS to reduce inflammation and thus relieve pain.

As far as specific impact on PD goes, the evidence is still a work in progress. I've read a couple of trials but the number of people treated is really too small to say with certainty that it is or isn't effective in dealing with many Parkinson's symptoms.

It looks very likely that medical cannabis is good for improving the quality of life of many patients. (Pain relief will do that.)

There are also strong indications that patients using the drug sleep better. Back in Chapter **2** you might recall that I mentioned Rapid eye movement Behaviour Disorder (RBD). I've seen one test report, with an admittedly small sample, that stated emphatically: "patients treated with cannabidiol had prompt and substantial reduction in the frequency of RBD-related events without side effects."[33]

Speaking of side effects, other studies have indicated that some people do experience some negative responses to cannabidiol. These have included nausea, diarrhoea, appetite changes (plus or minus), anxiety and drowsiness.

Please note: cannabidiol is *not* the stuff in marijuana that gets people high. That's a substance called THC – *tetrahydrocannibinol* if you want its full name. While it's a psychoactive drug, THC is thought to have some therapeutic value too. (It's also where a lot of the negative publicity comes from.) Some of the cannabis that's available for medical use has deliberately low levels of THC.

I've read interviews with patients who reckon the low-THC version is less effective in dealing with their symptoms. That might be true, or it might be because having become used to one reaction to treatment, they're just not willing to accept something different. There really doesn't seem to be enough evidence to make a statement either way, other than for an individual's own experience.

Based on those individual experiences and the weight of history there is a need for a lot more research to be done on the potential of medical marijuana. That's not easy in a political and social environment where the "anti-drug message" is sometimes more shrill than sensible. The abuse of cannabis is a problem, just like the abuse of a lot of other things. Controlled use is another matter. Study should trump emotion when there's such a strong prospect of making a positive difference in people's lives.

If you're given the opportunity to trial medical cannabis by your doctor, maybe as an oil or in capsule form, it's worth considering – particularly if you're in significant pain. Report back honestly please. Whether it works for you or not, your evidence can only help others – PD patients and more.

Simply put: There is some evidence that medical cannabis can help PD patients, particularly with pain relief and sleep disorders. More research is required.

---

*

5.8 Infra-red therapy

One of the newest options for PD patients to consider is *photobiomodulation*, or infra-red therapy, also called *NIr therapy*. It means shining a light on the brain, but a very particular light, and on very particular parts of the brain.

Infra-red radiation isn't visible to the human eye, although some commercial bits of equipment marketed as 'infrared' (e.g. some 'therapeutic' heat lamps) use a bulb that produces a red light to go with the heat they generate. But true infra-red does more than warm things up.

Radiation has some interesting effects on living cells. The negative ones are quite well known, and have been since not long after the a-bombs were dropped on Japan. But there are different kinds of radiation, and some of the effects can be positive.

The infra-red radiation used in NIr therapy for example apparently works to functionally repair damaged dopamine-producing cells deep in the brain. It won't replace those that have died off completely, but it does seem to improve the production and release of dopamine, which in turn means a reduction in the symptoms of PD.

This is another avenue that needs a lot more exploration. A lot of the testing that's happened so far has been done on monkeys, not humans. Their brains are similar, yes, but not quite the same. But there have been trials done on people too, and the results have been impressive.

One thing that's been learned is that the radiation works best at quite close range. So to be really effective, whatever is generating the radiation has to be as near as possible to the affected areas, deep in the brain.

That's the limitation on one of the 'delivery methods' sometimes offered – a device that looks a bit like a salon hair dryer, lowered over the patient's head. The infra-red rays have to get through hair, scalp, skull, and 80 – 100 millimetres of brain tissue to get to their target. The signal is really weak by the time it's done that, so while there's a certain amount of benefit to some parts of the brain that are affected by the loss of dopamine (and that benefit shows up in some symptomatic relief) it's not really getting to the main problem area for PD: the area that actually produces the dopamine[34].

There are two alternative solutions that I'm aware of. One (that I'm not aware of having been tried on human patients) is to surgically insert a tiny optical fibre device inside the brain as close as possible to the area most affected by the disease. So far the trials have been good, with clear signs of improvement in cell health and symptoms, and no sign of any harm being done to any of the surrounding tissues. It's worked well on rats, mice and monkeys. Another area of research that's a work in progress…

The other 'delivery method' that's showing promise is intra-nasal. A small device reminiscent of a pen torch gets inserted in a nostril and sends a dose of the infrared rays up into the brain. It's a shorter distance to the dopamine-producing cells, and there isn't a layer of skull in the way. Not as good as the optical fibre, but less invasive, it requires no surgery.

Such evidence as I've seen is mostly anecdotal, but I do know of PD patients who've reported a lot of improvement in their symptoms using the 'light up the nose'.

NIr therapy is not a 'one-off' treatment, but the effects seem to last longer the closer the radiation source is to the affected part of the brain. This is an important element of the research that still needs to be done.

Professor Simon Lewis, director of the PD Research Clinic at the Brain and Mind Centre in Sydney is cautious but positive about the work done so far on NIr therapy:

> "It's encouraging research, and in the absence of a cure we shouldn't disregard any suggestion, but we must strike a balance between hope and hype. The concern is that people might go out and buy a device which might be expensive, whereas in reality they may be better off spending money on proven therapies, such as exercise therapy or speech therapy, which are definitely going to help everybody with Parkinson's. (However) the bottom line is, there is very reasonable science behind infra-red light therapy, and I think we should be very open to conducting a well-constructed clinical trial."[35]

There's one especially encouraging thing about the infra-red therapy that's been studied thus far. According to Professor Jonathon Stone, the executive director of the Bosch Institute (the University of Sydney medical research centre), "it's so blessedly free of side-effects that you can use it without having to know down to the last molecular detail how it works."[36]

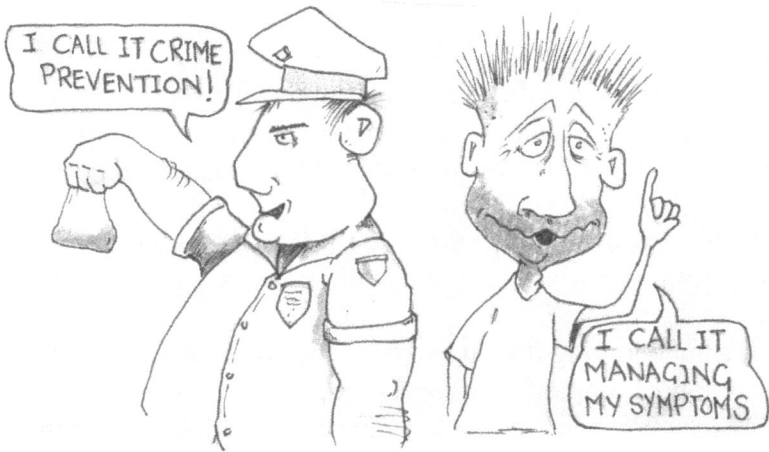

Good quality medical grade **cannabis** may be an effective treatment for some symptoms of Parkinson's Disease. (pg 49)

> **Simply put:** Infra-red therapy: directing particular wavelengths of light into the brain, shows promise in repairing the damaged cells responsible for PD. More research is definitely worth pursuing.

*

5.9 Feldenkrais

Alternative therapies attract a lot of debate. Many are dismissed by skeptics, but are defended passionately not only by their practitioners, but by patients who feel the therapy has done them real good.

It's the essence of faith healing – if you wholeheartedly *believe* that something will make you well, your brain overcomes what's going on with your body and allows it to heal itself. It's the positive side of the coin that says that if you keep declaring, "This'll never work", it won't.

The *Feldenkrais Method* is one such therapy, and it's one that presents itself as being of particular value to Parkinson's patients.

The Method takes its name from its founder – Dr. Moshe Feldenkrais. He was an engineer, physicist, inventor, martial artist and a student of human development (from anatomy and physiology to movement science and child psychology). He applied his studies and judo training to his own serious knee injury and was able to overcome the need for risky surgery.

That led him to develop an exercise therapy based on improving the relationship between movement and consciousness – repairing damaged connections between the body and the motor cortex. That's the part of the brain responsible for initiating and controlling voluntary movement. Feldenkrais practitioner Roger Bowden explains it this way:

"People often find that through these improvements, they become aware of further improvements in their overall health and well-being, leading to better attention, thinking ability, emotional resilience, coordination, balance and breathing.
Specifically for people with Parkinson's Disease, we look for improving flexibility and mobility, ability to remain more upright (prevent stooped posture), maintaining balance and step length, and prevention of falls."[37]

In a session, a Feldenkrais practitioner directs attention to habitual movement patterns that are thought to be inefficient or strained, and attempts to teach new patterns using gentle, slow, repeated movements. Slow repetition is believed to be necessary to impart a new habit and allow it to begin to feel normal. The patient might actively perform the specific actions, or the practitioner may be more 'hands on' in actually directing the movement.

The sessions may be 1:1, in which case the patient will sit or lie down on a padded table while the practitioner guides careful movements requiring as little effort as possible. He or she will touch precise points on the body to raise awareness in different areas. In a group session (sometimes called Awareness Through Movement classes) everyone is taken through a planned sequence of gentle movements, intended to let each person explore the range they're capable of. In particular, the idea is to pay attention to the sensations of the movements, not just in the part of the body that's in action, so that with practice the control gets 'hard-wired' back into the brain.

There is plenty of evidence that the brain is better than we thought at healing itself, if encouraged the right way. The term sometimes used is *neuroplasticity*. The Feldenkrais Method is about exploring, and tapping into that ability.

The biggest problem, and one that the skeptics and critics seize on, is a lack of hard scientific data to support Feldenkrais' claims. The small number of studies done haven't been especially rigorous. So much so that when the Australian government conducted a rigorous review of alternative therapies (assessing what should be eligible for health insurance subsidy), the Feldenkrais Method was one of seventeen that didn't 'make the cut'. The review said, "Overall, the effectiveness of Feldenkrais for the improvement of health outcomes in people with any clinical condition was felt to be uncertain."[38]

Skepticism and a lack of government support don't deter the Method's practitioners and supporters though. And to be fair, a lack of 'hard data' doesn't mean a therapy doesn't work – only that it hasn't been "conclusively proven".

Much of the most emphatic praise for Feldenkrais comes from people who swear that it's made a big positive difference to their lives, with comments like: "I always feel at the end of the class that my posture has improved. I can be standing more upright, or feel more grounded and evenly balanced on my feet."[39]

Simply put: Feldenkrais is a routine of gentle guided exercise that may be of value in improving the brain-to-body link in Parkinson's patients. Anecdotal evidence is good but there's been little scientific research.

---

*

5.10 Intentional Laughing

Not all forms of exercise feel like exercise. There's a lot more that can help besides the gym, and touching your toes and skipping.

It's also important to look for activities you can enjoy that *aren't* just Parkinson's-focused. After all, PD shouldn't define who you are or limit what you want to do. There are things you can do that are a.) enjoyable, and b.) helpful, not least because you're sharing the experience with other people who are enjoying themselves.

It may never have occurred to you, but laughing is really good for you. You breathe deeply, so lots of oxygen gets into your blood and your body, which is great for your muscles and organs including your brain. Speaking of the brain, laughter triggers production of endorphins and the release of seratonin, which is why a good bout of laughter leaves you feeling relaxed.

'Intentional laughter' isn't the same as going to watch a stand-up comedian or watching an old Jerry Lewis movie on DVD. You may not find either of them funny. Humour is subjective – I loved the *Goon Show* and cringed at *Funniest Home Videos*, my Mum had it the other way around.

But the funny thing is (excuse the pun) that your brain doesn't know the difference between real and 'fake' laughter. The oxygen still comes in, and the hormones and neurotransmitters still get produced.

An Intentional Laughter session (sometimes called Laughter Yoga – don't worry, it's because of the breathing, not because you have to tie your body into odd positions) isn't about telling jokes. It's about deep breathing, and going "Ha ha ha, ho ho ho," even if you don't feel like it. If it sounds weird and you reckon you'd feel like a dill, don't worry. When there are a few people all doing it together in a group session like a 'Laughter Club', it's amazing how quickly the forced fake laughter turns into the genuine article.

For someone with PD one of these sessions works on several levels at once: good chemistry in the brain to help improve mood and manage pain; increases oxygen; reduces stress (you really can't laugh and feel stressed at the same time); social interaction; and a fun way of being distracted from the condition for a while.

That social interaction in a positive, happy environment shouldn't be underestimated. It's unfortunately all too easy for people with a chronic condition like PD to make a 'shell' for themselves and withdraw into it. Sharing a laugh can be a good reminder that you're still part of the human race and you can enjoy other people's company – and they can enjoy yours.

Even so, Intentional Laughter can also be done in a 1:1 session with a trained practitioner, for someone who likes the idea but is a bit self-conscious about laughing in front of others at first. All the physical benefits are still there, and given time I reckon most people will want to share the experience with like-minded others.

The practice was developed in India in 1995, and has spread around the world quickly. Because it's not physically demanding it's good for people with movement and mobility issues. I've seen a film clip of a roomful of people hooked up to dialysis machines enjoying an Intentional Laughter session. Not just enjoying it, but according to the Deakin University report done at the time, getting the benefits of a significant reduction in episodes of intradialytic hypotension (sudden low blood pressure during dialysis), improved mood, enhanced optimism and decreased stress.[40]

Potentially the same benefits could be there for PD patients. Karen Flannery, a Laughter Leader, facilitator and teacher, told me of one of the 'regulars' at her weekly Laughter Club. This lady has quite severe Parkinson's, but found that laughter was improving her ability to cope with the condition – she was learning to laugh again and have fun in a safe environment. Her daughter came along as well, and could see the improvement. Sometimes the lady would arrive with her hands shaking severely, but by the end of the session she'd be safely fetching her own cup of tea!

Karen has also delivered an Intentional Laughter session to a Parkinson's Support Group (both patients and carers), and reports that there was a dramatic improvement of feelings in the room by the time she'd finished. They'd started out hesitant and uncertain, but ended up all smiles and chatting. Karen especially noticed one bloke in the front row who'd looked extremely stressed and unhappy when she began, but by the end was smiling broadly and keen for a chat. The change in his mood was obvious![41]

Intentional Laughter is another field that requires a lot more serious research. Studies have been done – I mentioned the one on dialysis patients, and a study has been conducted recently in Melbourne on the benefits of laughter for chronic pain patients. (I'm told the results were very promising but as I write this the report hasn't been released.) Whilst the research is still limited, the anecdotal evidence that I've seen is good. As with any therapy, what you'll get out of it will be driven in part by what you put in. At the very least, a session should be good for a laugh!

Simply put: Intentional laughter can offer a degree of both physical and psychological relief from some of the symptoms of Parkinson's.

*

5.11 Dancing

I've said repeatedly how important movement is in managing PD. One way of helping to make that movement happen is dance.

Now I'll be honest here. I'm no dancer. I can move roughly in time to music (I love music), but what I do is so uncoordinated and awkward that when I worked in musical theatre, despairing choreographers got me to stand still and let everyone else dance around me.

But that really doesn't matter. Even if your skills are on a par with mine, the activity of *trying* to dance can do you good. And it really doesn't matter what style you have a go at. Polka to pogo, break dance to barn dance, watusi to waltz – they're all about movement and rhythm.

I reckon that rhythm is the key to how it works. I read an interview with a PD patient in England who said that's what her body responds well to. Importantly, she says it's something she remembers when her body freezes (a common symptom) and she has trouble walking.[42]

While you could have a go at any dance class, it's worth noting that there are specifically designed programs called **Dance For PD**. These originated in collaboration between the Mark Morris Dance Company and the Brooklyn Parkinson Group in New York in 2001, and now the classes happen in thirty countries across the world. There are around thirty such classes taking place across Australia, so the opportunity may be closer than you think!

You don't have to be an accomplished or experienced dancer to begin with. You don't even have to be steady on your feet. Around half the class is conducted sitting down, and the remainder can be tailored to suit people whose lack of safe mobility confines them to a chair. Time and practice will hopefully help remedy that for them.

The idea is to engage both mind and body in a supportive social environment, and focus on artistic expression rather than emphasise the 'therapy' aspect. People in the classes are encouraged to approach their movement like dancers, not patients. It means boosting confidence, and transforming attitudes about living with a chronic condition ("Oh no, I couldn't do that... hey, wow! I just did!"). The interactions within the class help overcome the social isolation which can be a signpost to depression.

And while those psychological benefits are happening, there is some good physical stuff going on, too. The body and the brain respond to music as a reflex. It's why so many of us unconsciously tap a foot to a song on the radio, for instance. So when a dance instructor gently 'ties' a movement to the rhythm it reinforces a connection in the brain and improves control.

Philip Piggin is a dance practitioner in Canberra who leads Dance For PD classes from his base at Belconnen Arts Centre. He describes it this way:
> "It's extraordinary how the music sets up this whole neural pathway connection that seems to override the dyskinesia and freezing often experienced with Parkinson's. The dancers will often come in with a tremor or stoop, but when the music's on and they're moving, we see this lift. We're constantly encouraging them to lengthen their bodies and engage their abdominals, and we see them become more upright, animated and engaged with the wider world."[43]

The routine and rhythm of dance are also helpful in improving 'muscle sense'. A big part of dance practice is noticing and being aware of how the body is moving. As that awareness gets better, it can carry over into

61

other, more basic actions like walking and climbing stairs.

Those types of physical changes may not happen for everyone. Each patient's body is unique, and much may depend on their precise symptoms and how advanced the PD is. As with any such therapy, a good rule is 'no new pain'. But as long as it's comfortable, dance is a legitimate and effective form of exercise (I keep saying how important that is), and if it's one that you get pleasure from then I reckon it's well worth exploring.

> **Simply put:** Dance classes, and especially Dance For PD, offer social and psychological benefits for PD patients, and might also provide improvements in managing some physical symptoms.

*

5.12 Speech therapy and Singing

People with little or no first hand experience of Parkinson's tend to think of it as affecting the arms and legs. The unfortunate reality, as noted in **Chapter 2**, is that it can be a lot tougher than that. The face and particularly the jaw are often affected. It can be tremors in the jaw, or the awkward immobility sometimes called 'frozen face'. There can be trouble with any or all of the muscles in the larynx (voice box), throat, tongue, lips and the roof of the mouth. This can cause difficulty with both speaking and swallowing.

Speech is a particular problem for as many as half of all PD patients. The trouble is usually with any or all of volume, pronunciation, or prosody. (Prosody is defined as that aspect of spoken language which consists in correct placing of pitch and stress on syllables and words. It is responsible for conveying subtle changes of meaning, independently of words or grammatical order. You can tell prosody is impaired when the voice becomes flat and monotone.)

As with the other parts of the body, exercise can be really valuable in overcoming these symptoms. A study in Glasgow in the early 1980s showed two to three weeks of daily exercises emphasizing volume and tone not only significantly improved patients' speech, but that improvement was sustained for up to three months.[44]

Further studies over subsequent years have reinforced those findings. Results have been assessed both clinically (by recording and testing against 'benchmarks') and by consulting family, carers and close friends of the patients in the study.

Speech therapy can be delivered in a number of ways. One particular program that has been researched extensively and shown to get good results is the Lee Silverman Voice Therapy Program (LSVT). Named for the first patient for whom it was designed, this program is an intensive 1:1 treatment delivered over a month. For four weeks the patient attends four one-hour sessions per week, and every day completes a ten to fifteen minute set of vocal exercises as 'homework'. These home exercises then continue on after the clinical sessions to reinforce the work. The program is based largely on strengthening the voice box, and improving the patient's own awareness of the sounds they make. Definitely *not* about shouting! Each individual patient has their own program devised to address their own particular problems and issues.

Not every speech therapist can deliver the LSVT program – it requires specific training and accreditation. But as I said, there are other approaches that a professional in the industry might take. If your voice is starting to go, it could be well worth a consultation.

A less conventional therapeutic approach to helping with this problem area is *singing*. I mentioned at **5.11** above how helpful music can be. This is a logical extension of that. Singers do a whole range of warm-up exercises (not to mention the actual performance itself) that closely resemble things that a speech therapist would guide a patient through.

To explore this further, in May 2017 the Queensland Conservatorium of Music Research Centre and the Queensland Health Department launched a research project. Groups of PD patients in different parts of the world were taken through a weekly one-hour guided singing session for 24 weeks, with various measures of their quality of life being taken before, during and after the program.

According to the results released in February 2018 by Griffith University, singing made a measurable and overall positive difference to people with Parkinson's.

You might be one of the many people out there who reckons they can't sing. I've got a friend who couldn't carry a tune in a bucket. Doesn't matter! It's not about performing at the opera, or a blues festival, or getting onto a TV talent show. It's about rescuing your voice from deteriorating further, and improving the use of it. And about enjoying the experience.

Elizabeth Lord is a singing teacher who facilitated the Brisbane section of the research project I mentioned above, and who leads the 'Conquest Singers' – a choir of people with Parkinson's, and their carers. She says:
> "Being able to sing is optional, group singing is more about sharing and having fun in a positive atmosphere while keeping the moving parts of the voice well-oiled as we sing the songs we love. In this nurturing environment, surrounded by music, where we share time with others who understand some of what we may be going through, people may have the opportunity to experience a wide range of benefits that could have a positive effect on their physical, social an emotional wellbeing."[45]

Of course there are a lot of choirs and social singing groups out there, and many of them are really social gatherings who sing, rather than Serious Musicians (i.e. they care more about enthusiasm than the quality of someone's voice). Search on-line for who is in your area, or if you're old-fashioned like me, check the phone book.

If you have enough self-confidence to join a choir, or a bunch of 'performers' like a barbershop quartet, then go for it, I say! Or stay comfortable in a group that just sing for their own enjoyment, not anybody else's.

But it *is* encouraging to know that there are some PD-specific groups and programs starting to become available.

Simply put: both speech therapy and singing offer exercise that can help improve muscle control and PD symptoms around the mouth and throat. They can also offer some good social benefits.

---

*

5.13 Nutrition and diet

As you're probably aware, there are huge numbers of diets and dietary supplements out there, making all sorts of claims about an even bigger range of health benefits.

The link between what we eat and how our body behaves is pretty obvious. It shows up in things like food allergies, sugar levels in diabetics, even how some kids react to red cordial! Given how important nutrition is to overall health, it's not unreasonable to consider that Parkinson's, being a condition based on body chemistry, might respond (positively or negatively) to particular things that are eaten or drunk.

Yet there doesn't seem to have been a great deal of specific research done on the topic. Lots on diet in general, but not much that's particular to PD. The basic recommendation on just about every PD website is: "eat well, eat a balanced diet". Good advice, but it applies to pretty well everyone!

One study of over a thousand PD patients did offer a list of foods suggested to be linked to a reduced or more rapid progression of Parkinson's symptoms, although it didn't dig into *why* these foods gave the results. But the data is interesting.

Foods associated with a *reduced* rate of PD progression were: Fresh fruit & vegetables, nuts & seeds, non-fried fish, wine, olive oil, coconut oil, fresh herbs & spices.

Foods associated with *more rapid* PD progression were: Canned fruit & vegetables, soft drink (both diet and regular), fried food, beef, ice cream, yoghurt, cheese.[46]

The same study also looked at some supplements, and noted that *iron supplements* were associated with more rapid progression of symptoms, while *coenzyme Q10* (CoQ10) was associated with a reduced rate.

This CoQ10 is a nutrient that is naturally produced in a healthy body. It's an antioxidant that protects cells from damage. CoQ10 levels seem to be lower in PD patients, but whether that's 'cause' or 'effect' isn't clear. The nutrient is present in a lot of foods: heart, liver, kidneys, pork, beef, chicken, trout, herring, sardines, mackerel, spinach, cauliflower, broccoli, oranges, strawberries, soybeans, lentils and peanuts.

It's also increasingly common as a supplement in capsule form. A warning: not all supplements are created equal. Don't just look for the cheapest option (although price doesn't guarantee quality, either). One tip is to look for evidence of reputable, independent testing. Not just the endorsement of a sports star who's getting paid to push a product, but something like: "accredited by NSF International Dietary Supplement Verification Program" or "approved by the Australian Therapeutic Goods Authority".

You might have heard of probiotics, or seen them in the supermarket. They're products that boost the good bacteria living in your gut – the bacteria responsible for digesting your food properly and getting all the good stuff from that food into your system. Way back in **Chapter 1** I talked about the possibility of a link between the gut and PD. I've read a case study that trialled giving Parkinson's patients a daily dose of a probiotic every day for twelve weeks. Compared to the patients given only a placebo pill instead, those on the probiotics showed a "measurable improvement" in their symptoms at the end of the twelve weeks compared to before the trial. It's a good result, but it wasn't a big group and there was no further digging to determine *why* the results were so good. But as with all PD research, it helps.

Sodium – that stuff that makes up 40% of ordinary table salt – helps control the fluid balance of the cells in your body. That effectively controls the way that muscles and nerves work. So it makes sense that it's been found that some PD patients, particularly those with tremors and twitches, seem to have low levels of sodium in their blood.

That does *not* mean you should start putting a load of extra salt on everything you eat. There should be enough in the food you already eat, especially in pre-prepared meals, tinned and frozen foods etc. Read the labels – see how much salt actually gets put in during the manufacturing process. Adding a bit of extra salt on your plate is probably only necessary if you're mostly living on a diet of fresh food, and you don't already add it in the cooking process.

Adding a *small* amount of salt might be recommended if you suffer from low blood pressure, but for most people there really is plenty naturally occurring in our regular diet. Well, perhaps not 'naturally'. Most PD websites actually recommend that you cut down on salt intake, reflecting what's written in most health-related and diet-related websites overall.

It's something that can be affected by some of the PD drugs. So when you and your doctor are checking on possible side effects if you start a drug treatment, look for sodium levels in a blood test.

> **Simply put:** While there's not enough research yet to link any particular foods or supplements as being especially good or bad for PD patients, a good balanced diet can only help!

There is one 'eating program' in particular that has recently been getting some publicity as being potentially helpful for people with Parkinson's.

It's called the ***ketogenic diet***. It's high in fat, and low in both carbo-hydrates and protein (so lots of dairy products!). That means that instead of burning sugar for energy, someone on the diet is burning fats or 'ketone bodies'. People promoting the diet reckon this is more 'efficient' fuel.

It's been used for some years to treat epilepsy that doesn't respond to medication. Effectiveness in dealing with PD is still very much at a pre-clinical, research stage. There is study underway to investigate wheth-er the ketogenic diet could decrease the formation of the alpha-synuclein protein that's found in clumps in the brains of Parkinson's victims. (That's part of the post-mortem 'testing' for PD I mentioned back in **Chapter 1**.)

There's also some suggestion that since the ketogenic diet is low in protein, which interferes with the absorption of levodopa (the chemical that should convert to dopamine), some benefit could perhaps be derived from improving the amount of levodopa getting into the body, rather than a direct effect on the brain itself. There's not much to go on yet for PD patients.

There are anecdotal reports and one case study in which five volunteers followed a ketogenic diet for 28 days. Trial participants had an improve-ment in their ability to perform daily activities and their motor symptoms, but with such a small group there could be plenty of other things involved.

And like any 'special diet', it shouldn't be 'jumped into' without care and attention. It needs supervision by a doctor (and also, preferably, a dieti-cian). The potential side effects include dehydration, low glucose and kid-ney stones. It's a strict diet that can be tough to follow and could put you at risk for certain nutritional deficiencies, so if you try it you can expect regular blood tests to make sure your body has all that it needs.

Simply put: The ketogenic diet (high fat, low protein & low carbs) might have some value for PD patients, but needs to be tried under proper medical supervision.

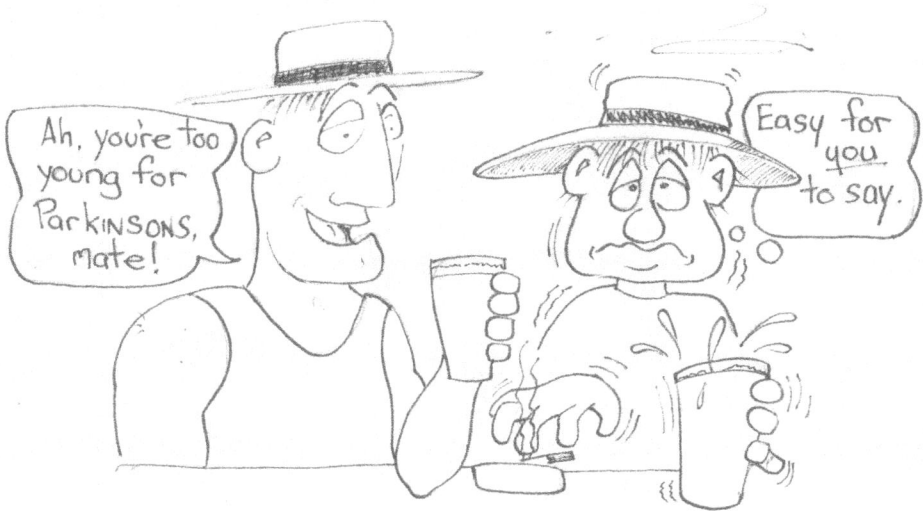

Parkinson's Disease may often not be **diagnosed**
until after the age of fifty, but that doesn't mean
it's not there. (pg 12)

6 WHAT CAN I DO FOR MYSELF?

Quite a few of the activities I've talked about in Chapter 5 aren't necessarily or always 'Parkinson's specific', and that's a good thing. The more
stuff you can do that's open to everyone, the less you define yourself as a
"person with Parkinson's". The *person* is more important than the disease.
Or put another way, you may have it, but it doesn't have you.

That attitude is important in getting on with your life.

I'm not suggesting that you be unrealistic and try to do stuff that's truly
physically beyond you. If you've never been a long-distance runner then
it's probably not the time to take on your first-ever marathon. Not without
a whole lot of working up to it. But that's the point - you *can* set achiev-
able goals for yourself and have a bloody good go at reaching them, one at
a time.

If you can walk, then do so. If a walk to the corner store is beyond you,
try doing a lap of the house. A gentle stroll out to the front garden and
back is better than a whole day sunk in an armchair watching daytime tele-
vision. Just do your best – the more 'best' you're capable of, the more you
should try. You might just find that when you push yourself a little you'll
get more good results than you expected.

A positive attitude alone won't always be enough to get you better. Sometimes the body needs help, from whatever source. But a negative attitude
will stop any attempt at improving from being successful.

The mother of a friend of mine had a fall, and convinced herself her legs
would never work again. Weeks later she was physically fine – back,
legs, bones, muscles, nerves all fully healed – but she couldn't walk. No
amount of drugs, physiotherapy, chiropractic work, hypnotherapy or
meditation helped, because she steadfastly didn't *believe* they'd help. She
spent the rest of a miserable existence levering herself between a wheel-
chair, an armchair, and mostly, her bed.

70

If you convince yourself that you're "only going to get worse" then that's EXACTLY what will happen. No matter what therapy, drugs or activity you try, the PD will take you on a steadily downward course.

But I hope over the preceding pages I've shown you that there are ways to slow down, maybe even stop the gradual deterioration. And the fundamental key to that outcome is movement. Regular, repetitive, and mindful.

It's also important to remember that, no matter how down you may be feeling, you are *not alone*! There are **support groups** for people with Parkinson's. These are made up of other patients and carers, who share their experiences both bad and (most importantly) positive.

Some of them are active social groups, involved in going out and *doing* things together. Things like walking, laughing, singing, and dancing. Others are more inclined to sit around and chat over a cup of tea, or even a beer, about what's working for them.

Any activity is good, both for the sake of movement and for the social connection. Being alone is one thing – some blokes really enjoy their own company. But *loneliness* is perhaps the worst feeling a person can suffer. And very often PD can lead someone into that terrible feeling of isolation.

Even if what you find is a very low-key group who just sit around and talk about how they feel, just being part of a conversation can help. There's an old saying: a burden shared must become lighter.

Please try to avoid making it a 'race to the bottom'. "Oh, *my* symptoms are so much worse than yours..." Comments like that don't help anyone, although I'm sure you'll hear them sometimes. (Misery loves company is another old saying.)

But you can at least compare what you've tried, what you've done this week that's new, whether it worked or not. Someone else might be inspired to try for themselves, or warned off if it proved to be an especially bad idea.

Search on-line. Check your local phone book. Check out the notice boards in the shopping centre. Talk to your doctor.

If there seems to be nothing organized near where you live, could you be the one to start it? Put up an ad on that notice board, or just explain to the doc that you'd like to get together with other folks in the same position as you. If he or she is really any good as a doctor they'll do what they can to support the idea, even if it's just talking to those other patients and giving out whatever contact details you're willing to share. Even an on-line community is better than feeling isolated, although nothing beats real human company.

Simply put: your best chance of living well with Parkinson's is to be as active as you can, be positive about the things you do, and accept (and offer) company and support.

.o0o.

7 A QUIET WORD TO CARERS

It's not easy to be the person who 'looks after' a Parkinson's patient. That's especially true if you're pretty much the "sole carer". There are physical, psychological and emotional challenges so it's important that you take care of your own health in all of these areas.

There's a good reason why airlines always tell passengers: "In case of emergency fit your own oxygen mask before assisting others".

Unfortunately, 'burn out' is all too common among care givers, and those looking after PD patients are every bit as at risk as people looking after the sufferers of any other debilitating condition. Try to be aware of how you're feeling. It's natural to be tired, but constantly exhausted is too much. Having moments of feeling overwhelmed is understandable, but if that's how you feel most (or worse, all) of the time then you need to do something about it.

In **Chapter 6** I talked about *support groups*. They're just as important for a carer as they are for the person with Parkinson's. They remind you that you're not alone, and can allow you to let loose some of your fears, frustrations and concerns among people who best understand what you're going through.

They offer positive experiences too. People can share tips and advice you hadn't thought of or heard about. Coping tips for both you and the person you look after. The simple pleasure of social interaction – eye contact with somebody different – can be really uplifting for someone who feels like the world has shrunk to revolve around just one other person.

Here are a few other things that might be a part of the role you find yourself in. Many of them you probably already know, but if I can offer any fresh advice, tips or a different perspective that can help, then I'll be pleased:

Be prepared to *expand the medical team*. Add as many experts and opinions you can to the group that are offering potential solutions. As well as a good General Practitioner look out for specialists: Consultant Physicians, physiotherapists, exercise physiologists, dieticians – specialists in any or all of the things discussed in **Chapter 5** and any more that you discover.

If they're not talking to each other already, then you can help by conveying information from one to another. They may not always agree with each other. That's okay – as long as they are aware of what they're each recommending, and you and the patient are keeping a watchful eye on proceedings. In some ways you're the eyes and ears of the medical team, because you see the patient more regularly, and more closely, than anyone. This may not get said as often as it should, but believe me – you're appreciated!

The more you can *stay organized* the better it will be for everyone, including you. It's a big help in reducing your own stress if you can find what works best for you for keeping track of things.

You might need to know what medications need to be taken and when. That's the sort of thing that can be written down and displayed somewhere prominent. Writing these things down and keeping them visible is helpful for your memory (and the patient's) and invaluable to anyone who may be assisting you for the first time or at short notice.

Likewise use a calendar, or a large visible diary for appointments, both the regular and occasional ones. Not just doctors', but whatever classes and fun things you might do together. The same goes for keeping tabs of when a prescription needs to be filled or renewed.

I suggest you include your own appointments, because it's all too easy to lose focus when you're concentrating on someone else. Don't forget or skip your own important stuff because you're 'too busy' with the person you're caring for.

Stay informed. Reading this book is a help (thank you!) but also keep an eye and ear out for other sources of information and advice. Doctors' waiting rooms, the library, the newspaper, even the internet can offer something useful. Don't just take it at face value though – ask questions and look for second opinions and confirmations.

Education is really valuable for you. Learn what you can about PD and its symptoms. The more you know about what's going on with your loved one, and what may happen in the future, the more chance you have of coping with it. It will never be easy, but dealing with the unknown is worse. Getting caught off guard can really unbalance you. If a boxer sees a punch coming, even if he can't dodge it he can brace for it. It's the blow you don't expect that does the most damage.

The more you learn, the more you may be able to help the person you're caring for, too. You can't make someone try a treatment that they don't want to. Well, maybe you can, but under those circumstances it's a LOT less likely to work. But the more you know, good and bad, the more you can put a reasonable case for them to give it a go.

Something that often lurks in the shadows behind Parkinson's is *depression*. It can strike the patient, and it can also hit you. As much as possible, be aware of their moods and your own. Feeling down from time to time is entirely understandable under the circumstances you're both in, but sometimes a line gets crossed and you really need to ask for professional help.

Here are some of the 'clinical' signs of depression. If you notice any number of these becoming regular (or worse, constant!) it's definitely time to look for support:
- angry outbursts;
- appetite changes;
- sleep problems;
- anxiety;
- agitation;
- problems with reasoning ;
- failure to recognise or engage with familiar people and things.

Normally you'd start by talking to your, or their, doctor. In an emergency though, remember that there are 'help lines' dedicated to just such crises.

Here are some resources I know of, but you should always check locally and make sure you've got useful contact information somewhere handy.

<u>Australia</u>	Beyond Blue 1300 224636
	Lifeline 13 11 14
	www.lifeline.org.au/Get-Help/Online-services/crisis-chat
<u>USA</u>	Samaritans (212) 673-3000
	NDMDA Depression hotline 800-826-3632
<u>UK</u>	Samaritans 0845 790 9090
	www.depressionuk.org

Depression, yours or someone else's, is never something you should try to battle alone. I know, I've been there. That's why I'm so glad that there are organisations, and people, ready and willing to help.

Lastly I'll repeat: *look after yourself.* You can't look after others if you don't take care of yourself. Eat properly. Exercise regularly, even if it's just going for a quiet walk. Get all the sleep you can.

Figure out what helps you to de-stress. Maybe it's sport, or writing, or yoga. Colouring in, reading, meditation, swimming laps, riding your bike – any or all can help, whatever works for you is what's right, so try until you finds what makes you feel better.

And build a support network. Find friends or family members who can step in when you need a break, even if only for an hour or two. Investigate respite care: there are organisations that specialise in it, and there may be support available to help you get it. Even a few days off can make a great positive difference for you, and the better shape you're in, the better you can be at caring for someone else.

Never forget, even if it may not be expressed as well or as often as it might or should be in some cases, *you are appreciated!*

.o0o.

CONCLUSION:

THE FUTURE FOR PARKINSON'S

A lot of modern medicine is about fixing or easing symptoms. Yes, that *is* important, especially for the poor sod suffering. But the real key is addressing the problem *behind* the symptoms.

Imagine you've got a car that keeps getting dents in the bodywork from big hard pinecones falling from the tree you park under every day. You could ignore the dents until rust gets in and the car falls apart. You could go to the panel beater regularly and get the dents knocked out. That's fixing the symptoms. Or you could get the dents knocked out once, and then park somewhere else, or build a carport, or even cut down the tree (sorry green people – not my preferred option!). That's addressing the cause of the problem.

The only way that can happen with Parkinson's, or any other disease for that matter, is through research. There *is* a lot of that being done, all over the world. You might have noticed that in this book – I've been reading and referring to a lot of it and I know there's plenty more out there.

You can do something to support that research! I don't necessarily mean financially, though that always helps. But *talk* to people. Talk to doctors, tell them what you're going through, good and bad. What's working and what isn't.

Good researchers talk to doctors and get their input, drawing on their experience and the experiences of their patients. Every case study is another piece of evidence. Get involved in clinical trials if you have the chance. That's where we get what knowledge we have.

That's the way in which someone, somewhere in the future, hopefully not too distant, is going to work out how to cure Parkinson's. Or even prevent it. It'll take a combination of
- time,

- patience,
- commitment,
- study,

and crucially, the input of people who are living with the condition but willing to help.

I'm confident that a cure is in the future, and not too far away. I look at the number of other diseases that have been overcome during my lifetime – yes, lots haven't, but there is progress being made, and the work being done now on PD is definitely looking promising. Already there are ways to make lives easier and symptoms more bearable.

Your own future though is in your own hands. Sitting on them won't help. Get up, get out, and get going. Move that body – and move it like you mean it!

.xXx.

FOOTNOTES

1   McCallum, Katie *Muhammad Ali's Advocacy for Parkinson's Disease Endures with Boxing Legacy*, parkinsonsnewstoday.com June 10, 2016

2   Heyn, Sietske N. & Charles Patrick Davis *Parkinson's disease: Symptoms, Signs, Causes, Stages and Treatments*, medicine.net January 1, 2018

3   Stefanis, Leonidas *Alpha-Synuclein in Parkinson's Disease*, Cold Springs Harbor Perspectives in Medicine, February 2012

4   Mehanna, Raja et al *Comparing clinical features of young onset, middle onset and late onset Parkinson's Disease*, Parkinsonism and Related Disorders Journal, Vol 20, Issue 5, May 2014

5   McDermott, Annette & Alana Biggers MD MPH, *Early Onset Parkinson's Disease*, healthline.com, 30 November 2016

6   Stern, Matthew B. *Head Trauma As A Risk Factor For Parkinson's Disease*, Movement Disorders Journal, Volume 6 Issue 2, 1991

7   Nixon, Jeff *NFL Concussion Settlement: How did the NFL underestimate the prevalence of Parkinson's disease?* sportsblog.com, 19 May 2018

8   Bakalar, Nicholas *Concussions May Increase the Risk for Parkinson's Disease*, New York Times, 18 April, 2018

9   Nield, David *We Just Got More New Evidence That Parkinson's Starts in The Gut - Not The Brain,* sciencealert.com 28 April 2017

10   Svensson, Elisabeth PhD et al *Vagotomy and subsequent risk of Parkinson's disease*, Annals of Neurology, published online June 2015

11   Svensson, *ibid*

12   Bojing Liu cited in Neild, *op cit*

13   Ahiskog, J. Eric PhD, MD *The New Parkinson's Disease Treatment Book (Second Edition)* Oxford University Press, New York, 2015

14   Heyn & Davis, *op cit*

15   Case-Lo, Christine & Graham Rogers MD *Symptoms of Parkinson's: Men vs. Women*, healthline.com 15 August, 2016

16   Case-Lo, *ibid*

17   Downward, Emily *Parkinson's Disease in Men*, parkinsonsdisease.net March 2017

18   Case-Lo, *op cit*

19   Paparrigopoulos, Thomas J. *REM sleep behaviour disorder: Clinical profiles and pathophysiology*, International Review of Psychiatry Volume 17, 2005 – Issue 4

20   Downward, *op cit*

21   Heyn & Davis, *op cit*

22   Sherman, Brian with A.M. Jonson *The Lives of Brian,* MUP 2018

23   Konczak, Professor Juergen, *personal comment*, September 2018

24   Cooper, Professor Matt, *Australian Parkinson's Research Makes Exciting Discovery*, cited by Shake It Up Australia Foundation, shakeitup.org.au, 7 November 2018

25   American Society of Exercise Physiologists *Definition of Exercise Physiology*, asep.org, undated

26   McConaghy, Melissa, quoted in *Targeted neuro-physiotherapy intervention vital in effective management of Parkinson's disease*, physiotherapy.asn.au 12 April, 2018

27   Mukherjee, Bipasha *A Cure for Parkinson's disease?* modernreflexology.com Undated 2018

28   Zukerman, Wendy *Chinese medicine offers new Parkinson's treatments*, newscientist.com 17 June 2011

29   Yeo, Sujung et al *Neuroprotective Changes of Thalamic Degeneration-Related Gene Expression by Acupuncture in an MPTP Mouse Model of Parkinsonism: Microarray Analysis*, Gene 9 December 2012, cited in healthcmi.com

30   Yeo et al, *ibid*

31   Lee, Sook-Hyun & Sabina Lim *Clinical effectiveness of acupuncture on Parkinson disease*, Medicine (Baltimore) Volume 96(3) January 2017

32   Wang , Fang et al *Effect and Potential Mechanism of Electroacupuncture Add-On Treatment in Patients with Parkinson's Disease* Evidence-Based Complementary and Alternative Medicine, Volume 2015, Article ID 692795, 15 March 2015

33   Chagas, M. H. et al *Cannabidiol can improve complex sleep-related behaviours*, Journal of Clinical Pharm Therapy Epub 21 May, 2014

34   Johnstone, Daniel M. et al *Turning On Lights to Stop Neurodegeneration*, Frontiers In Neuroscience 11 January, 2016

35   Lewis quoted in Suvi Mahonen *Let There Be Light*, The Weekend Australian Magazine, 7 October 2017

36   Stone quoted in Mahonen, *ibid*

37   Bowden, Roger *Feldenkrais*, moveit4parkinsons.com.au, August 2018

38   Gavura, Scott *Australian review finds no benefit to 17 natural therapies*, sciencebasedmedicine.org, 19 November 2015

39   S. Williams quoted in *Feldenkrais*, moveit4parkinsons.com.au, August 2018

40   Bennett, Paul N. et al *Intradialytic Laughter Yoga therapy for hae-modialysis patients: a pre-post intervention feasibility study*, BMC Complementary and Alternative Medicine Journal 15:176, 9 June 2015

41   Flannery, Karen *– personal comment*, November 2018

42   Mitchell, Melissa *Dance brings patients together* physiotherapy. asn.au July 16, 2018

43   Piggin, Philip - *personal comment*, September 2018

44   Scott, Sheila *Speech therapy for Parkinson's disease*, Journal of Neurology, Neurosurgery, and Psychiatry 46:140-144, 1983

45   Lord, Elizabeth quoted in *Singing for Parkinson's*, moveit4parkinsons.com.au August 2018

46   Mischley L. K., R. C. Lau & R. D. Bennett *Role of Diet and Nutritional Supplements in Parkinson's Disease Progression*, Oxidative Medicine and Cellular Longevity 2017: 6405278, Epub 10 September 2017

GLOSSARY

(Here are some words and terms you may hear or read in connection with Parkinson's, including in this book. I've tried to explain in as simple terms as I could. This is taken, and expanded, from the Glossary on the excellent website parkinsonsvic.org.au . My sincere thanks to Parkinson's Victoria.)

Acupuncture channels: (*jing luo* in Chinese) Also called meridians, a network of 12 main and 8 secondary pathways within the body along which energy (*qi*) flows between organs and under the skin. There may be 2000 acupuncture points along these channels.

Agonist: A substance that acts like another substance and therefore stimulates an action. So a 'dopamine agonist' is a drug that produces the same effects as naturally occuring dopamine.

Alpha-synuclein: A protein found in unusually large quantities in Lewy bodies, found in the brains of deceased PD patients. Researchers are looking at how it affects dopamine production, and whether it has a genetic link.

Apomine® (apomorphine hydrochloride): A dopamine agonist that's quick acting and is effective for a short duration. It is given by injection or continuous pump. Does NOT contain morphine.

Atypical Parkinsonism: Conditions that resemble Parkinson's but have some variations in symptoms and their response to medications that normally impact PD.

Basal Ganglia: A set of structures deep within the brain, that consists of the striatum, globus pallidus, subthalamic nucleus and substantia nigra. Dopamine is produced in the cells of the substantia nigra. The basal ganglia has important implications in movement, cognitive and emotional functions. It's this area that provides a definite diagnosis of Parkinson's, but unfortunately can only be properly examined in a post mortem.

Bradykinesia: Slowness in initiating and executing movement. One of the more common symptoms of Parkinson's.

Bradyphrenia: Slowness of thought process. A less common but distressing symptom of Parkinson's although more commonly associated with other conditions.

Cannabidiol: A key component of medicinal cannabis, thought to be useful in relieving chronic pain.

Carbidopa: A drug that prevents levodopa from being broken down before it reaches the brain, as it normally could be.

COMT Inhibitors (Catecholamine O-methyl Transferase): Contain an enzyme that prevents further breakdown of levodopa and extends the duration of the drug's effectiveness. Usually used as part of a combination therapy of levodopa, carbidopa and entacapone.

Coenzyme Q10 (CoQ10): A nutrient that naturally occurs in the body, acts as an antioxidant protecting against cell damage. CoQ10 levels are often reduced in PD patients.

DaTscan: A medical imaging technique that captures pictures of the dopamine system in the brain.

Deep Brain Stimulation (DBS): A reversible surgical procedure used in the management of Parkinson's. It involves placing electrodes into a chosen target site of the brain. This site choice depends on the aspect of Parkinson's to be treated – for example tremor, dyskinesia or bradykinesia. The electrodes are connected to a small generator that produces electrical impulses to manage the particular symptom.

Dopamine: A chemical produced by the substantia nigra in the basal ganglia. It is responsible for transmission of signals between nerve cells that control movement. A lack of dopamine is the primary factor in Parkinson's. The exact reason for this depletion of dopamine remains unknown but is the subject of much research!

Duodopa® (levodopa and carbidopa): A gel formulation of <u>Sinemet®</u> that's delivered via a permanent tube into the small intestine. This is an alternative mode of treatment in later stage Parkinson's.

Dysarthria: Difficulty speaking, in PD may be caused by problems with tremor or freezing of muscles of the mouth and jaw.

Dyskinesia: Involuntary movements (nodding, jerking, twisting). May be a symptom of PD, but may also result from medium to long-term use of <u>levodopa</u>.

Dysphagia: Difficulty swallowing, can be caused by problems with the muscles of the throat, or the tongue.

Dystonia: Sustained posturing (i.e. 'stuck' in an uncomfortable and/or abnormal position) that can affect any part of the body, more commonly seen in the feet, toes and neck.

Endorphins: Chemicals produced within the brain that affect the nervous system, reducing the perception of pain, in a similar way to drugs like morphine and codiene. Sometimes called the 'pleasure hormones'.

Entacapone: A <u>COMT inhibitor</u> used in combination with other medicines to treat the '<u>wearing off</u>' of <u>levodopa</u> treatment. It inhibits enzymes that would otherwise break down levodopa.

Freezing: The temporary inability to move. Freezing may only last a few seconds. It can occur in confined spaces or when changing direction. An occasional symptom of PD, also associated with other physical and psychological conditions.

GB34 (He-Sea, earth point, heavenly star point): A point on the 'Gall bladder <u>acupuncture channel</u>' commonly used for the treatment of tendon, ligament and joint disorders, and pain related conditions such as sciatica, hip pain, joint pain, muscle pain, tendon pain and knee pain.

Gou teng: A herb with hook-like branches used in Chinese medicine. It's believed to reduce <u>alpha-synuclein</u> clusters without harming the immune system.

Idiopathic: A term meaning 'cause unknown', usually applied to any disease or condition that appears spontaneously for no apparent reason.

Infra-red Therapy: Also called NIr Therapy or photomodulation. A treatment that involves applying infra-red light to parts of the brain, intended to affect the production of dopamine.

Kampavata: An ancient (5000 B.C.) name for what we now call Parkinson's.

Kinson® (levodopa and carbidopa): A dopamine replacement therapy medication. Not usually called an agonist because it's a compound of two substances.

Kripton® (bromocriptine mesylate): A dopamine agonist medication.

Levodopa (L-dopa): A chemical precursor of dopamine that can be taken orally. It is converted to dopamine and crosses the blood brain barrier. It occurs naturally in some plants and is now also made synthetically.

Lewy Bodies: Round microscopic structures found in brain cells, often regarded as a definitive sign of Idiopathic Parkinson's. Unfortunately, they're usually only found at a post-mortem.

Liquid Sinemet® (levodopa and carbidopa): A liquid preparation of Sinemet® that's made up daily and taken every one or two hours. It may be prescribed in complex cases of Parkinson's.

LV3 (sometimes called Great Rushing or Taichong): A point on the 'Liver acupuncture channel' commonly used for the treatment of menstrual disorders, headaches, dizziness, epilepsy, high blood pressure, insomnia, blurry vision and tremors, making it especially important in the treatment of PD.

Madopar® (levodopa and benserazide): A dopamine replacement therapy medication available in rapid, normal and controlled release preparations. Not usually described as an agonist because it's a compound of substances.

MAOIs (Monoamine Oxidase Inhibitors) (Selegiline®, Elde-pryl®): Drugs that block the breakdown of dopamine in the brain. Drug interactions are possible with this group of medications.

Motor Fluctuations: A broad description of different responses to levodopa therapy that may develop after a few years of treatment. They may include 'wearing off', or 'on/off' phenomena. In addition to motor fluctuations, other symptoms may appear or fluctuate, including sweating, anxiety and pain.

Multiple System Atrophy (MSA): A relatively rare disorder that in its early stages can closely resemble, and sometimes be associated with Parkinson's. It involves progressive deterioration and death of different types of nerve cells in the brain and spinal cord.

Neupro® (rotigotine): A dopamine agonist administered via a patch worn on the skin. The patch is changed daily and should be refrigerated before use.

NIr Therapy: See Infra-red Therapy.

'On-Off' Phenomena: Motor fluctuations resulting from medium to long term use of levodopa. Usually refers to the patient's original symptoms suddenly recurring, sometimes in short bursts. This can be abrupt and unpredictable.

Orthostatic hypotension: Uncharacteristically low blood pressure when you stand up, or remain upright for any length of time.

Pallidotomy: A surgical procedure in which the globus pallidus region of the brain is deliberately scarred in an effort to lessen Parkinson's symptoms.

Parkinsonism/Parkinsonian: Conditions that resemble Parkinson's because of the symptoms e.g. the presence of muscle rigidity, tremor, and bradykinesia, but may be caused by something other than a dopamine problem. These are also known as atypical Parkinsonism or pseudo-Parkinsonism.

Parkinsonian gait: A distinctive shuffling walk, often stooped, with reduced or no arm swing and difficulty balancing.

Parkinson's Plus: A group of conditions that make up other forms of progressive Parkinsonism. These include Multiple System Atrophy (MSA) and Progressive Supranuclear Palsy (PSP).

Parlodel® (bromocriptine): A dopamine agonist medication.

Permax® (pergolide mesylate): A dopamine agonist medication.

Pill-rolling: A term sometimes used for the symptom more usually called tremor.

Progressive Supranuclear Palsy (PSP): A comparatively rare degenerative disease that damages nerve cells in the brain. Many symptoms are common to Parkinson's, but PSP particularly affects eye movement, resulting in blurred vision.

Rapamycin: A drug used to suppress tissue rejection in transplant patients, potentially valuable for PD patients in removing alpha-synuclein clusters, but with a high risk of compromising the immune system.

Rapid Eye Movement Behaviour Disorder (RBD): Normally, a sleeping person has no muscle tone and doesn't move during sleep. In RBD, a person can move limbs and seem to act out their dreams.

Remedial massage: Also called therapeutic massage, it's meant to relieve or assist with a specific medical issue. As distinct from 'relaxation' massage.

Resting Tremor: A tremor that occurs when the affected limb or body part is at rest (not necessarily during sleep). Can be exacerbated with stress.

Restless Legs Syndrome: A sensory disorder that commonly occurs in Parkinson's patients but is actually not related to PD. It's characterised by the urge to move the legs either during sleep or awake at rest.

Rigidity: This is when muscles feel stiff and inflexible rigidity during passive movement (e.g. when your arms swing while you're walking). It may be associated with tremor, but not necessarily.

Selgene® (selegiline hydrochloride): Refer to MAOIs (monoamine oxidase inhibitors).

Seratonin: A compound in the blood that acts to constrict the blood vessels. It is believed to help regulate mood and social behaviour, appetite and digestion, sleep, memory, and sexual desire and function.

Sifrol® (pramipexole): A dopamine agonist medication.

Sinemet® (levodopa and carbidopa): A dopamine replacement therapy medication available in normal and controlled release. Liquid Sinemet® can be prepared from this medication.

Stalevo® (Catecholamine O-methyl Transferase (COMT) Inhibitors): Contains an enzyme that prevents further breakdown and extends the duration of the effectiveness of levodopa. It is a combination therapy of levodopa, carbidopa and entacapone.

Striatum: A part of the basal ganglia, responsible for transmitting dopamine from the substantia nigra to the rest of the basal ganglia, making it a key part of the control of voluntary movement.

Substantia Nigra: This is the deepest structure within the basal ganglia, and is located around the top of the spine in the brain stem. Dopamine is produced in the substantia nigra and sends signals from there up to the striatum. A loss of dopamine producing cells within the substantia nigra is the primary cause of Parkinson's symptoms.

Symmetrel® (amantadine): An anti-viral medication that's thought to increase dopamine release in the brain and therefore may be used in the treatment of Parkinson's.

Tasmar® (tolcapone): This original COMT inhibitor is no longer widely used due to the risk of hepatic failure.

Thalamotomy: A surgical procedure, now less commonly performed than it once was, in which brain cells in the thalamus are destroyed in an effort to eradicate debilitating tremors.

Therapeutic massage: See <u>Remedial massage</u>.

Tremor: An involuntary rhythmic movement that usually occurs when the affected body part is not in use or at rest. It may affect any part of the body but predominantly occurs in the upper or lower limbs or jaw and is often initially seen on one side of the body. Internal tremor may be felt but is not visible. Not all cases of Parkinson's will experience tremor.

Ubiquinone: Another name for the antioxidant nutrient <u>CoQuinone 10</u>.

Wearing Off: A variance in response to <u>levodopa</u> therapy that may develop after a few years of treatment. Basically, whatever relief had previously been achieved gets less, or even disappears completely. See <u>motor fluctuations</u>.

REFERENCES

Ahiskog, J. Eric PhD, MD *The New Parkinson's Disease Treatment Book (Second Edition)* Oxford University Press, New York, 2015

Aman, J., A. Abosch, M. Bebler, C. Lu & J. Kanczak *Subthalmic nucleus deep brain stimulation improves somosensory function in Parkinson's disease* Movement Disorders: Journal of the Movement Disorder Society Feb 2014 29(2):221-8, epub 15 November 2013

American Parkinson Disease Association *Early Onset Parkinson's Disease*, apdaparkinson.org, undated

American Society of Exercise Physiologists *Definition of Exercise Physiology*, asep.org, undated

Association of Traditional Chinese Medicine & Acupuncture UK *Scalp Acupuncture Treatment for Parkinson's Disease*, atcm.co.uk 2015

Australian Physiotherapy Association *What is physio?* physiotherapy.asn.au, undated

Bakalar, Nicholas *Concussions May Increase the Risk for Parkinson's Disease*, New York Times, 18 April, 2018

Baricheila, M. et al *Dietary habits and neurological features of Parkinson's disease patients: Implications for practice*, Clinical Nutrition 36 (4) 1054-1061, August 2017

Bennett, Paul N. et al *Intradialytic Laughter Yoga therapy for haemodialysis patients: a pre-post intervention feasibility study*, BMC Complementary and Alternative Medicine Journal 15:176, 9 June 2015

Bowden, Roger *Feldenkrais*, moveit4parkinsons.com.au, August 2018

Calvert, Robert Noah *The History of Massage*, Healing Arts Press, Vermont, 2002

Case-Lo, Christine & Graham Rogers MD *Symptoms of Parkinson's: Men vs. Women*, healthline.com 15 August, 2016

Chagas M. H. et al *Cannabidiol can improve complex sleep-related behaviours*, Journal of Clinical Pharm Therapy Epub 21 May, 2014

Chagas M. H. et al *Effects of cannabidiol in the treatment of patients with Parkinson's disease: an exploratory double-blind trial*, Journal of Psychopharmacology Epub 18 September, 2014

Chaudhry, Uzma & Lee Kieft *Apomorphine Information Sheet*, Parkinson's UK, March 2018

Cleveland Clinic *Speech Therapy for Parkinson's Disease*, my.clevelandclinic.org 6 October 2014

Cooper, Professor Matt *Australian Parkinson's Research Makes Exciting Discovery*, cited by Shake It Up Australia Foundation, shakeitup.org.au, 7 November 2018

Dolhun, Rachel MD *Head Trauma and Parkinson's Disease*, michaeljfox.org 17 June, 2016

Dolhun, Rachel MD *What's the best diet for Parkinson's?* michaeljfox.org 27 July, 2017

Downward, Emily *Parkinson's Disease in Men*, parkinsonsdisease.net March 2017

Duvoisin, Roger C. & Jacob Sage *Parkinson's Disease: A Guide for Patient and Family*, Lippincott Williams & Wilkins, New Jersey, 2001

Dwyer, Julie *Targeted neuro-physiotherapy intervention vital in effective management of Parkinson's disease*, physiotherapy.asn.au 12 April, 2018

Flannery, Karen, Laughter Leader, Facilitator and Teacher, Hervey Bay, Queensland, *personal comment*, November 2018

Gasior, Maciej, Michael A. Rogawski & Adam L. Hartman *Neuroprotective and disease-modifying effects of the ketogenic diet*, Behavioral Pharmacology September 2006

Gavura, Scott *Australian review finds no benefit to 17 natural therapies*, sciencebasedmedicine.org, 19 November 2015

Gordon, Richard et al *Inflammasome inhibition prevents a-synuclein pathology and dopaminergic neurodegeneration in mice*, Science Translational Medicine Vol. 10 Issue 465, 31 October 2018

Heyn, Sietske N. & Charles Patrick Davis *Parkinson's disease: Symptoms, Signs, Causes, Stages and Treatments*, medicine.net 1 January, 2018

Iffland, Kerstin & Franjo Grotenhermen *An Update on Safety and Side Effects of Cannabidiol: A Review of Clinical Data and Relevant Animal Studies*, Cannabis Cannabinoid Research 2017 Epub 1 June, 2017

Jacobs J. V. & F. B. Horak *Abnormal Proprioceptive-Motor Integration Contributes To Hypometric Postural Responses of Subjects With Parkinson's Disease* Neuroscience 141 (2006) 999-1009, 14 April 2006

Johnson J. A. & T. R. Pring *Speech therapy and Parkinson's disease: A review and further data*, British Journal of Disorders of Communication Volume 25 1990, Issue 2

Johnstone, Daniel M. et al *Turning On Lights to Stop Neurodegeneration*, Frontiers In Neuroscience 11 January, 2016

Knaster, Mirka *Discovering the Body's Wisdom: A Comprehensive Guide to More Than Fifty Mind-Body Practices*, Bantam 1996

Konczak, Juergen, Director, Center for Clinical Movement Science, University of Minnesota, *personal comment*, September 2018

Konczak, Juergen et al *Proprioception and Motor Control in Parkinson's Disease* Journal of Motor Behaviour Vol. 41 No. 6, 29 May 2009

Kubala, Jillian MS, RD *7 Benefits and Uses of CBD Oil (Plus Side Effects)* healthline.com/nutrition 26 February, 2018

lee, Sook-Hyun & Sabina Lim *Clinical effectiveness of acupuncture on Parkinson disease*, Medicine (Baltimore) Volume 96(3) January 2017

Levine, Andrew *The Bodywork and Massage Sourcebook*, Lowell House 1998

Loria, Kevin *11 key findings from one of the most comprehensive reports ever on the health effects of marijuana*, cannabis-md.com 1 February, 2017

Lev, N. & E. Melamed *Heredity in Parkinson's Disease: new findings*, Israel Medical Association Journal June 2001

LSVT Global *What is LSVT LOUD treatment?* lsvtglobal.com 2018

Maguire, Emily *Ketogenic Diet and Parkinson's Disease,* ketodietapp.com 4 April, 2017

Mahonen, Suvi *Let There Be Light*, The Weekend Australian Magazine 7 October, 2017

Mandal, Dr Ananya MD *Parkinson's Disease History*, news-medical.net 24 January, 2013

Mao, Cheng-jie et al *Serum sodium and chloride are inversely associated with dyskinesia in Parkinson's disease patients*, Brain Behaviour e00867, 9 November 2017

McCallum, Katie *Muhammad Ali's Advocacy for Parkinson's Disease Endures with Boxing Legacy*, parkinsonsnewstoday.com 10 June, 2016

McDermott, Annette & Alana Biggers MD MPH, *Early Onset Parkinson's Disease*, healthline.com 30 November, 2016

Mehanna, Raja et al *Comparing clinical features of young onset, middle onset and late onset Parkinson's Disease*, Parkinsonism and Related Disorders Journal, Vol 20, Issue 5, May 2014

Mischley, L. K., R. C. Lau & R. D. Bennett *Role of Diet and Nutritional Supplements in Parkinson's Disease Progression*, Oxidative Medicine and Cellular Longevity 2017: 6405278, Epub 10 September 2017

Mouslech, Z. & V. Valla *Endocannabinoid system: An overview of its potential in current medical practice*, Neuro Endocrinol Letters 2009: 30(2): 153-79

Mukherjee, Bipasha *A Cure for Parkinson's disease?* modernreflexology.com Undated 2018

Neuroscience Research Australia, Dr. Scott Kim & Dr. Nicolas Dzamko *Parkinson's disease and related syndromes* neura.edu.au Undated 2018

Nichols, Hannah *Everything you need to know about estrogen*, medicalnewstoday.com 2 January, 2018

Nield, David *We Just Got More New Evidence That Parkinson's Starts in The Gut - Not The Brain,* sciencealert.com 28 April, 2017

Nixon, Jeff *NFL Concussion Settlement: How did the NFL underestimate the prevalence of Parkinson's disease?* sportsblog.com 19 May, 2018

O'Suilleabhain, P., J. Bullard & R. B. Dewey *Proprioception in Parkinson's disease is acutely depressed by dopaminergic medications* Journal of Neurology, Neurosurgery & Psychiatry 2001, 71:607-610, 26 June 2001

Paparrigopoulos, Thomas J. *REM sleep behaviour disorder: Clinical profiles and pathophysiology*, International Review of Psychiatry Volume 17, 2005 – Issue 4

Piggin, Philip, Dance for PD practitioner, Belconnen Arts Centre *personal comment* September 2018

Samara, Denholm *Restorative dance promotes wellbeing*, Canberra Weekly

Scott, Sheila *Speech therapy for Parkinson's disease*, Journal of Neurology, Neurosurgery, and Psychiatry 46:140-144, 1983

Sherman, Brian with A.M. Jonson *The Lives of Brian,* MUP 2018

Smallridge, Jennifer *Difference between a physiotherapist and an exercise physiologist?* upwellhealth.com.au 23 June, 2018

Stalker, D. & C. Gylmour (eds.) *Examining Holistic Medicine*, Prometheus 1989

Stefanis, Leonidas *Alpha-Synuclein in Parkinson's Disease*, Cold Springs Harbor Perspectives in Medicine, February 2012

Stern, Matthew B. *Head Trauma As A Risk Factor For Parkinson's Disease*, Movement Disorders Journal, Volume 6 Issue 2, 1991

Stewart, D. O. et al *Prior history of head trauma in Parkinson's Disease*, Movement Disorders Journal, Volume 6 Issue 3, 1991

Svensson, Elisabeth PhD et al *Vagotomy and subsequent risk of Parkinson's disease*, Annals of Neurology, published online June 2015

Tamtaji, O. R. et al *Clinical and metabolic response to probiotic administration in people with Parkinson's disease: A randomized, double-blind, placebo-controlled trial*, Clinical Nutrition in ncbi.nlm.nih.gov, 1 June 2018

Wang, Fang et al *Effect and Potential Mechanism of Electroacupuncture Add-On Treatment in Patients with Parkinson's Disease* Evidence-Based Complementary and Alternative Medicine, Volume 2015, Article ID 692795, 15 March 2015

Wattanathorn, Jintanaporn & Chatchada Sutalangka *Laser Acupuncture at HT7 Acupoint Improves Cognitive Deficit, Neuronal Loss, Oxidative Stress, and Functions of Cholinergic and Dopaminergic Systems in Animal Model of Parkinson's Disease*, Evidence-Based Complementary and Alternative Medicine, Volume 2014 Article ID 937601, 5 August 2014

Yan, Yu, Traditional Chinese Medicine practitioner, Stratford-On-Avon *personal comment*, July 2018

Yeo, Sujung et al *Neuroprotective Changes of Thalamic Degeneration-Related Gene Expression by Acupuncture in an MPTP Mouse Model of Parkinsonism: Microarray Analysis*, Gene 9 December 2012, cited in healthcmi.com

Zeise-Suess, Dorothea GP *Treating Parkinson's Disease with Scalp Acupuncture*, parkinsonweb.com, August 2017

Zukerman, Wendy *Chinese medicine offers new Parkinson's treatments*, newscientist.com 17 June, 2011

Deep Brain Stimulation michaeljfox.org

Parkinson's Disease History parkinsons.org 23 June, 2009

ACKNOWLEDGEMENTS

There are, of course, a lot of people I must thank for their advice and assistance and input.

For starters, there's the team involved in the creation of the moveit4parkinsons website – a great resource for PD patients and their carers living in the NSW Northern Rivers region of Australia. The site, and their work, provided the initial inspiration for this book.

Many thanks to my own medical team, especially Hamish Lunn, Murray Parr, Warren Hirst and Nicola Cook. They've done a lot to keep me able to keep writing.

When I put out a call for some help with research Richard and Michelle Lum were quick to answer, and I'm very grateful.

Likewise, I'm very glad of the advice I've received from Dr. Bill Meyers on Queensland's Sunshine Coast, and Yu Yan (Jack) and Paige Du in the UK. They're authorities in their fields of expertise, and I am always grateful for their suggestions and input.

Professor Jeurgen Konczak at the University of Minnesota has been generous with his advice too, and I really appreciate the assistance of a gentleman of his authority in the medical profession.

I've had great support from the Laughter Yoga community in Australia and Japan. Special thanks go to Karen Flannery and Merv Neal for their insights and input.

I must also credit Sheila Zhou, Associate Scientist in the Australian Technical Services area of USANA Health Science. Sheila never tried to push her company's products, but with strict neutrality pointed me in the direction of some excellent, valuable research. From my own personal experience, I will just say that I've benefitted considerably from the USANA range.

Thanks again to Angus Gardner. We started knocking out cartoons together more years ago than either of us probably care to admit, and I still love his work!

I've enjoyed terrific love and support from Maggie Wildblood, a gifted writer herself. Maggie has consistently encouraged me to make my writing the best that it can be, and I hope I've lived up to her standards!

Finally, my last and greatest acknowledgement goes to my darling bride Meredith Yardley who really does put the 'courage' into encouraging me. While being passionate about Intentional Laughter, Meredith is really passionate about helping to improve people's lives in whatever ways we can. I doubt that I'd have started this book without her, far less finished it!

Thank you for reading - I sincerely hope that I've been able to offer some help, and perhaps more importantly some hope.

Now it's up to you.

www.ingramcontent.com/pod-product-compliance
Lightning Source LLC
Chambersburg PA
CBHW071115030426
42336CB00013BA/2087